Suffering in Paradise

Medieval & Renaissance Literary Studies

Suffering in
Paradise

The Bubonic Plague in English Literature from More to Milton

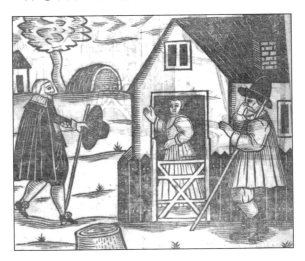

Rebecca Totaro

Duquesne University Press
Pittsburgh, Pa.

Published in the United States of America by

Duquesne University Press
600 Forbes Avenue
Pittsburgh, Pennsylvania 15282

Library of Congress Cataloging-in-Publication Data

Totaro, Rebecca Carol Noel, 1968–
    Suffering in paradise : the bubonic plague in English literature from More to Milton / by Rebecca Totaro.
        p. cm. — (Medieval & Renaissance literary studies)
    Includes bibliographical references and index.
    ISBN 0-8207-0362-1 (hardcover : alk. paper)
    1. English literature — Early modern, 1500–1700 — History and criticism. 2. Plague in literature. 3. Literature and medicine — England — History — 17th century. 4. Literature and medicine — England — History 16th century. 5. Plague — Great Britain — History. 6. Medicine in literature. 7. Diseases in literature. I. Title. II. Medieval and Renaissance literary studies
    PR408.P62T68 2005
    820.9'3561—dc22

                                                          2004024178

∞ Printed on acid-free paper.

*For my parents, Michael John and
Martha Jean Totaro, with love and gratitude*

Contents

Illustrations

Acknowledgments

The idea for this project originated in conversations with Charlotte Spivack at the University of Massachusetts, Amherst, in 1994. It became clear that Shakespeare's plays were riddled with plague language previously unstudied. Further research indicated that the prose and poetry of the period were infused as well and that writers addressing utopia in some fashion, regardless of the genre or stance, had consistently included the bubonic plague in their works. From there, under the direction of Wally Kerrigan, and with guidance from Charlotte, Kirby Farrell, Daniel Gordon (in the Department of History) and Arthur Kinney, the study flourished. Over the next six years, Wally held the bar high, and the result was a crucial transformation in my reading, reasoning, writing and general comprehension of the research process. A travel grant from the university enabled me to present at the Society for Utopian Studies conference, where the work earned the 1997 Arthur O. Lewis Award for best paper by a junior scholar. Over the years, I have grown to appreciate the level of collegial yet rigorous exchange in the society, and it has been my privilege to serve on their steering and awards committees. At Florida Gulf Coast University, I have benefited from university travel grants, funding from the Division of Humanities and Arts, exceptional interlibrary loan guidance from Roberta Russell, and encouragement from colleagues. I owe a particular debt of gratitude to S. Gregory Tolley, professor of marine science, whose knowledge of history and science, love of literature, and skill as an editor show within these pages.

With respect to abiding intellectual exchange in this area of study, I am most indebted to Lyman Tower Sargent (University of Missouri, St. Louis), Carrie Hintz (Queens College, CUNY), and Wendy Furman-Adams (Whittier College). Since 1998, Lyman has mentored me in the field of utopian studies and in the pursuit of serious scholarship. He read various parts of this manuscript before bringing his expertise to bear on the whole — a whole already profiting from his indispensable work in the field. Where there is style herein, this I largely owe to Carrie. With patience and wit, she taught me Publishing 101, read the manuscript in full, and helped me to recast it into a more seamless whole. If there is spirit, I attribute it to Wendy, who has offered inspiration and advice since 1989. She taught me by example that joy and good storytelling can transform labor into something sublime — especially when Milton is involved.

Portions of this book were published previously. Part of the introduction appeared in "English Plague and New World Promise," *Utopian Studies* 10, no. 1 (1999): 1–12. A lengthier version of chapter 3 appeared in "Bubonic Plague in *Utopia* and Old World Implications," *Q/W/E/R/T/Y: Arts, Litteratures, and Civilizations du Monde Anglophone* 8 (October 1998): 67–88. Part of chapter 7 appeared in "'Fly from that Pestilent Destruction': Plague in the Works of Margaret Cavendish," *In-between: Essays and Studies in Literary Criticism* 9, no. 1 (2000): 107–16. For permission to reprint, I owe thanks to the editors: Lyman Tower Sargent, Bertrand Rouge, and G. R. Taneja, respectively. Finally, I close with appreciation for Albert C. Labriola, Susan Wadsworth-Booth, Kathleen Meyer, Sandra Boatwright, and the editorial board at Duquesne University Press, whose excellent communication and high expectations have conspired to make this part of the process creative and rewarding.

Introduction

From its first visitation in 1348 to well after its last in 1666, the bubonic plague inhabited England and the lives of her citizens. No one escaped its threat. No one could imagine immunity. All modified their lives to make room for its presence and to control it on literal and conceptual levels. During times of increased mortality, those who could afford to flee from infected cities left livelihood and home behind. Those unable or unwilling to abandon their posts stayed to witness the red crosses on doors, the tolling of bells, and plague cart collections. During these times, the clergy debated the effectiveness of prayer and whether or not flight from plague indicated lack of trust in God. The devoted reconsidered their faiths. Monarchs terminated or delayed meetings of parliament. They issued proclamations in an effort to control its spread, and they followed their doctors and clergymen in flight from the infected capital. Dramatists depended on performing in the country or writing poetry during London visitations as they reconsidered their career options. Plague forced doctors to examine their own practices as well, pushing some to experiment, many to frustration, and a few to martyrdom. All trade became suspect, when it did not come to a standstill. Even the sight of a letter could cause alarm. The pattern of visitation was never quite regular enough for citizens to develop habits of survival that might seem somehow normal; one never knew when the plague would visit or how long it would last. In their abrupt departures from seats of government and in royal proclamations intended to control everything from religious ritual to trade and dietary habits, the kings and queens of early modern England left a particularly clear record of fear and of action. They had good reason to do so.

The bubonic plague threatened the security of each reign and of each royal lineage. Like a Shakespearean Richard III, waiting for a time of prosperity to seize the crown and initiate a reign of terror, the plague haunted the English throne. When it did not lurk in the background, it leapt to the stage of London and forced kings and queens to flee. In essence, it took over as the head of the nation, serving forcibly in the following periods:

Henry VII (1485–1509):   1498, 1504, 1505, 1509
Henry VIII (1509–1547):   1511–1521, 1523, 1535, 1543
Elizabeth I (1558–1603):   1563–1564, 1592–1593, 1603
James I (1603–1625):   1603–1611
Charles I (1625–1649):   1625–1626, 1636–1638, 1638–1639,
                            1641, 1643–1647
Charles II (1660–1685):   1664–1666

These plague years reflect the highest spikes in a chart of mortality rates derived from parish registers, but they also mark the years when plague ruled the minds of the nation and inscribed itself in literature.[1]

Even when mortality rates remained normal, the plague circulated its threat by rumors traveling across land and sea. Daniel Defoe's *Journal of the Plague Year* exemplifies the degree to which those rumors kept plague in power over lives, cities, nations, and narratives. In 1720 it struck France with enormous force, killing an estimated 50,000 in Marseille alone. Daniel Defoe wrote *Journal of the Plague Year* in 1722 as a warning to England to prepare for the worst. In it, the narrator

H.F. provides what is reputedly a firsthand and objective account of London's prior visitation in 1666. H.F. acts as the witness whom the reader can trust. By sharing his own story, he provides advice for those who will have to decide whether or not to flee from London during what Defoe and others believed was an impending visitation. H.F. had chosen to remain within the infected city, but by the end of the account, he assures readers that the horror of being trapped in the city warrants flight: "Upon the foot of all these Observations, I must say, that tho' Providence seem'd to direct my Conduct to be otherwise; yet it is my opinion, and I must leave it as a Prescription, (viz.) *that the best Physick against the Plague is to run away from it.*"[2] H.F. had made the wrong decision and is determined to spare others from doing the same. His description of people and of their struggle for survival under quarantine would convince any reader to flee when given the choice. So convincing was his depiction that it helped bring about the repeal of England's rigid 1721 Quarantine Act.

But when Defoe wrote *The Journal* and when Queen Anne issued the revised and softened Quarantine Act in 1722, plague had not visited England for over 60 years. The threat alone was enough to warrant action. Every rumor of plague suggested that England might again suffer, as it had repeatedly, as long as its inhabitants could remember. More specifically, we know now that the route of transmission from France to England was simple and common, taking only a few infected rats stowing away in a cargo hold. Early modern English men and women did not know that it was the *Yersinia pestis* bacteria that infected fleas who bit and infected them, but they did know the plague route. Rumors of plague in France and the Low Countries often preceded a London visitation. Defoe and others, including the queen, decided not to take any chances. They would prescribe the best methods available to them for preventing plague.

No other force in the period controlled the nation to such an extent. Only this enemy could force kings and queens to work around its schedule. In such times, the king or queen served as its pawn, and the English people saw their God-appointed sovereigns run. Under such conditions, a court page or cook breaking out in a fever was of concern enough to shake the national foundation, as Oxford writing master John Davies of Hereford explains in *Humours heau'n on earth with the ciuile warres of death and fortune. As also the triumph of death: or, the picture of the plague, according to the life; as it was in anno Domini 1603*:

> The King himselfe (O wretched Times the while!)
> From place to place, to save himselfe did flie,
> Which from himselfe himselfe did seeke t'exile,
> Who (as amaz'd) not safe, knew where to lie.
> Its hard with Subjects when the Soveraigne
> Hath no place free from plagues, his head to hide;
> And hardly can we say the King doth raigne,
> That no where, for just feare, can well abide.
> For, no where comes He but Death follows him
> Hard at the Heeles, and reacheth at his head.[3]

When plague took the throne, the king had "no place . . . his head to hide." The illustration on the frontispiece of Thomas Dekker's 1625 publication of *A Rod For Run-awayes* shows death as this inescapable tyrant, with all citizens forced to react (see figure 1). This was no way to keep a monarchy intact or society stable, and everyone knew it. They would have to construct a safe "no place" if they wanted a stable nation.

For these reasons, I refer to the period of plague in England, from the first visitation in 1348 to its last murmur in the first quarter of the eighteenth century, as "plague-time." Within this long period, the bubonic plague visited particular cities with increased force, so that one can refer to the particular visitation of 1603 or 1666, or the consecutive visitations of 1603–1611. Wartime would come and go, kings and queens

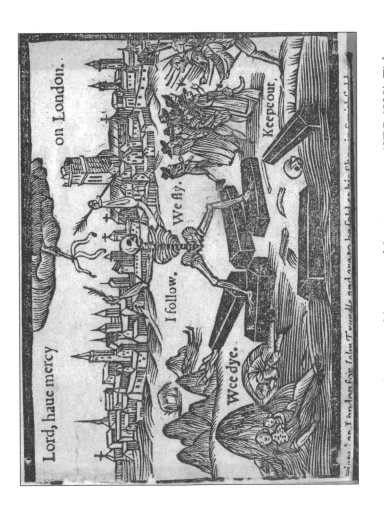

Figure 1. From Thomas Dekker, *A Rod for Run-awayes* (STC 6520). Title page. By permission of the Huntington Library.

would begin and end their reigns, famine and flood and fire would touch lives and then leave for decades. None of these things remained annually threatening over the course of centuries, ever in mind when not literally within bodies.

Yet, while we might easily consider plague as a constitutive force within early modern culture and therefore of the lived experience of all men, women, and children of the time, few studies of plague in early modern cultural or literary studies treat it as such. In the majority of scholarly examinations, plague is either a biographical or historical mile marker, or one of many physical afflictions more generally troubling early modern England. Both approaches deny the pervasive force of bubonic plague. The only book-length studies to focus on bubonic plague in early modern English literature, for example, treat it as one of many producers of cultural anxiety. In *To Blight With Plague: Studies in a Literary Theme* (1992), Barbara Fass Leavy covers literature from the late Middle Ages to the present and diseases from bubonic plague to AIDS. She discusses the general relationship between epidemics and the literary responses to them, which in her study are social and psychological at base. In *Fictions of Disease in Early Modern England: Bodies, Plagues, and Politics* (2001), Margaret Healy examines writings on bubonic plague, syphilis, and gluttonous behavior, concluding that they reveal social and psychological conceptions of embodiment that are at once like our own and foreign to them. Even Byron Lee Grigsby's *Pestilence in Medieval and Early Modern English Literature* (2004) treats bubonic plague alongside leprosy and syphilis, examining the degree to which the perception of each disease is a social construct.[4] These authors contribute to the study of bubonic plague, but in each study, bubonic plague becomes one of many frightful physical conditions utilized conceptually in order to register other concerns.

When we turn to early modern biographies written in the last decade, we find "plague" in the index with several corresponding pages listed.[5] Yet even so, almost every biographer to mention plague employs it as a catchy transition into a new chapter or in order to make claims regarding the physical whereabouts or financial situation of the person in question. Rarely do we read about the larger effect of plague on the author's life, on the way the author understood life, or on his or her works. For example, everyone studying early modern drama knows that during London visitations, kings and queens commanded the Privy Council to close the playhouses. Dramatists took their productions on the road and in some cases they supplemented their incomes by other means. But this is where the examination of plague most often ends.

There are a few exceptions, and to my knowledge, all exist in the area of Shakespeare studies, where biographies still garner enough of a readership that publishers can afford to produce them regularly. These exceptions include Leeds Barroll's *Politics, Plague, and Shakespeare's Theater: The Stuart Years* and Katherine Duncan-Jones's chapter "Plague and Poetry" in *Ungentle Shakespeare*. Barroll and Duncan-Jones deftly track Shakespeare's production rate for the plays and poetry, respectively, through a series of plague visitations. Barroll suggests that plague all but halted Shakespeare's production whenever the Privy Council closed the theaters. As soon as plague abated and Shakespeare was free to perform at the Globe, he began to write with noteworthy speed.

Barroll's larger claim is that Shakespeare's plays emerge "as crucial signifiers of cultural trauma."[6] The bubonic plague was one of the most potent sources of that trauma, it is relatively easy to mark, and therefore it stands reliably as a measure against which to read the plays. Rather than read Shakespeare's play-producing years as a seamless narrative of creativity, Barroll provides an alternative that admits realistic rifts. Katherine Duncan-Jones agrees: "Plague was a defining context for all Shakespeare's writing."[7] Both Barroll and Duncan-Jones use the timeline of plague visitations and theater closings to determine Shakespeare's literal whereabouts as well as his sources of income during those times. By doing so, they demonstrate that cultural anxieties influence lives and products, and they help to repair what Barroll, in 1991, saw as a problem within Shakespeare studies: "it is as if there were two separate conceptual entities: the dramatist, and his plays" (4). Some study lives. Some study works. Barroll and Duncan-Jones demonstrate why our own scholarly undertakings will be more complete and accurate if we unite these two conceptual entities.

We can extend this conclusion to all writers in plague-time. In terms of production rate and financial security, manuscripts were often delayed at the printer for fear of sending them through the mail. Writers often became more productive in the isolation of a country home when they fled the city. Patrons became either more or less generous in plague-time. Each of these things directly influenced writers' productivity and livelihoods, and each helped to determine writers' quality of life and, by extension, their conceptions of the human condition.

All lives — including those of the most imaginative of English writers — had a conceptual place for plague. And if all lives had a place for plague, then its influence reached beyond the politics and the cash flow of production. It crept into church sermons, into medical treatises, into royal proclamations, and into literary lives, cities, and worlds — the fabric of characters and plot and setting. Some of these plague-infected works display overt symptoms, and others ooze the odor of plague-time. Another set defiantly masks the buboes in their narratives in order to avoid detection, while others point out the sores of their readers; another group will stand determined to face the plague head on, in the hope of healing. Narrative content was not granted immunity from the threat inherent in the culture any more than kings, queens, clergymen, or commoners were.

Still, very few have examined the literal disease of the bubonic plague as a pervasive force in a play, prose work, or poem. Perhaps we have assumed that we should let the biographers and archivists note the mile markers of plague so that we can dutifully record the facts without having to think too much about them. Our reading of plague visitations has been a reading of static events. Instead plague must be read as a process at work in the lives of humans — one subject to interpretation by them as they wrote and by us, in retrospect, as we study their writings. Margaret Cavendish's *The Blazing World* is an interesting case in point. Cavendish, the Duchess of Newcastle, and her husband had returned to England from exile in France during the Interregnum. The return coincided not only with the Restoration of Charles II but also with what many call "The Great Plague" of London in 1666. Prior to the onslaught that year, Cavendish and her husband were living in London. To avoid the plague, they left to their country home. Soon thereafter she published her utopian romance. In this work, Cavendish includes a lengthy dialogue on the cause of the bubonic plague. Yet scholarly studies of the work focus almost exclusively on issues related to politics and feminism, with an occasional nod to natural philosophy as it serves one of the former discussions. There is so little scholarly treatment of plague in *The Blazing World* as to suggest it does not exist at all. A similar case can be made for examining *Romeo and Juliet*, *Timon of Athens*, Jonson's *The Alchemist*, or Milton's *Paradise Lost*. Each text bears within it the symptoms of an author living in plague-time. By examining the very plague-ridden content of each, we can better understand the period, the writer, and the content itself.

In order to compare these narratives forged in plague-time, we turn to plague as a common text — one that was read and interpreted by all in the period. There, within the narrative of the bubonic plague, men and women read of the literal manifestations of a horrible disease. They also found within it their own understandings of the body, of the human relationship with nature, and of the degree to which they had faith in their nation and their God. They found within it their limitations and their greatest potential.

An early modern writer's reading of the plague shows us in detail what he or she believes to be the parameters within which life as a human being occurs. These parameters are marked in various ways, but for now we can focus on the boldest boundaries of hope and despair. In plague-time, despair is an automatic response that fills poetry, plays, and prose. We see this in the refrain, "Lord, have mercy on us. Weep, fast, and pray," repeated time and again in prose pamphlets and woodcuts, as on the cover of T.B.'s 1625 *The Weeping Lady, or London Like Ninivie in Sack-Cloth* (see figure 2). But despair's sister is hope, an equally potent twin. To illustrate this, we can look to the production of literature itself. Quite simply, the literature produced at the time is itself a symptom of the hope forged out of plague-time — a hope identical to that borne out within parish birth records.

Births increased after each major visitation of the plague, and, like children born in the year following any war, they represent their parents' conviction that the future can be better. All parents generally hope that their children will see a more prosperous future, but each parent has very particular categories to fulfill. Some might wish their children better educated, more happily married, financially more secure, able to practice the religion of their choice without fear of punishment, or able to have sons in addition to daughters. Those having children in wartime might wish them a lifetime of peace. Those experiencing famine would wish for one without hunger. But all in plague-time would wish for better health. All in that period would hope that one day someone would find the cure for plague and for all physical ailments. This plague-induced wish helped to shape the dreams and the behavior of all parents in England for nearly 400 years.

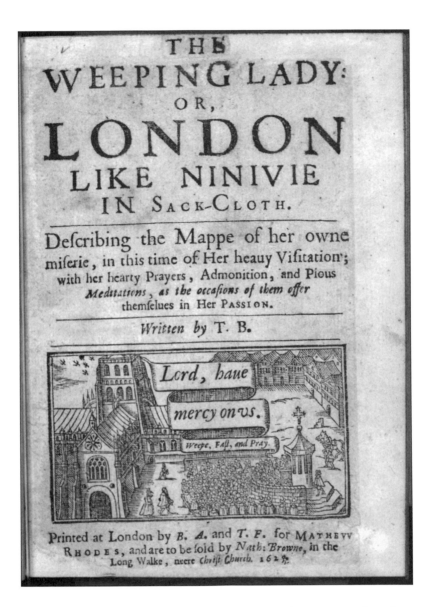

THE
WEEPING LADY:
OR,
LONDON
LIKE NINIVIE
IN SACK-CLOTH.

Deſcribing the Mappe of her owne
miſerie, in this time of Her heauy Viſitation;
with her hearty Prayers, Admonition, and Pious
Meditations, as the occaſions of them offer
themſelues in Her PASSION.

Written by T. B.

Lord, haue
mercy on vs.
Weepe, Faſt, and Pray.

Printed at London by B. A. and T. F. for Mathew
Rhodes, and are to be ſold by Nath: Browne, in the
Long Walke, neere Chriſt Church. 1625.

Figure 2. Thomas Brewer, *The Weeping Lady* (STC 3722). Title
page. By permission of the Huntington Library.

While many were busy wishing and living, others determined to put their plans for ideal health into writing. To do so, they first had to determine their relationship to bubonic plague, the most obvious gauge of life's limits. However, there were roadblocks around which none of the most visionary minds of the period would or perhaps could go. First, of course, was their lack of knowledge regarding bacteria, but if you were to supply them with such knowledge, they would still have found it difficult to maneuver around the Bible. A manual for plague prevention, the Bible was the primary comfort book for those afflicted. Doctors, preachers, average citizens, writers, and the monarchy alike learned from the Bible that with the Fall of Adam and Eve, sin became an inherent part of the human condition. With the seed of sin was sown disease, the inherent sin of the body and mind and the cause of its various issues — those oozy leakings, discolorations, deformities, and even mood swings.

The problem with taking action against pestilence in any form other than that determined by the church originated within the Old Testament interpretation of plague as God's rod of judgment. Created to correct the disobedient, gentile and Jew alike, the plague quite simply worked. God used it again and again and again, the best weapon in his cache. Furthermore, it appeared that God had decreed throughout the Bible — in Genesis, Exodus, Deuteronomy, Psalms, and through the prophets Jeremiah, Hosea, and Zechariah — that failing to acknowledge and uphold his law would lead directly to a plague visitation. This is in fact the origin of our word "plague." The Latin *plaga*, meaning to strike or blow, does not differ much from the term "scourge."[8] Once dispatched, God's blow could easily level an entire population. God alone might choose to relent, to spare his people from potential genocide, but although God promised Noah that there would be no future flood, God never removed plague from his arsenal of scourges. The early modern paradigm for the human

condition had a permanent place for plague and no one —
writer, doctor, king, or priest — was able to think beyond it.

One had to think with it, and it is not surprising to find
new genres of literature emerging to address this need. I refer
to these literary efforts as "plague literature": works produced
either in direct response to a plague visitation or those in which
bubonic plague functions as an essential event or primary
metaphor. For example, in his sonnets to Laura, who died of
the plague in 1348, Petrarch employs meter and rhyme to bring
her back in almost bodily form and free from signs of illness.
His sonnets, and those written in imitation for hundreds of
years afterward, owe their creation to plague as much as to
Petrarch. In the *Decameron*, Boccaccio wrote of a group of
men and women who move themselves beyond the reach of
plague. In a castle outside of infected Florence, they gather to
tell each other stories and thereby preserve their spirits and
their health. Plague initiated these tales, which in turn inspired Chaucer and many others. Prominent literary works
that have shaped a powerful canon for centuries, Petrarch's
sonnets and Boccaccio's tales are part of a yet-uncharted genre
of plague literature that spans generations and cultures.
Others writers contributed to the canon of plague literature
by imagining entire realms all but free from plague — a
virtual paradise in which suffering is kept to a minimum.

It is by examining these more complete visions of freedom
from plague that we can map out an increasingly realistic
course for hope in plague-time. *Mandeville's Travels* is a particularly interesting starting point. Sir John Mandeville published his *Travels* in Switzerland just nine years after the first
worldwide visitation of plague. Immediately successful, the
work was translated into nine languages within 100 years of
that initial publication in 1357. In England, the manuscript
circulated in at least five distinct English versions, accompanying the French and Latin. During the reign of Henry VII
alone, four separate editions were published. We also know

that Marco Polo, among others, relied on Mandeville to interpret his own experience at sea.[9]

In the *Travels*, Mandeville details his venture from England
to Constantinople, Jerusalem, and lands teeming with odd
inhabitants, before finally describing the famous Land of
Prester John where all inhabitants live in harmony. While its
validity was contested, even during his lifetime, *Mandeville's
Travels* appealed to a wide range of people over the course of
centuries. Mandeville's account of an island called Bragman
and its inhabitants must have been particularly attractive in
plague-time:

> Because they were so true and so rightful and so full of all good
> conditions, they were never grieved with tempests neither with
> thunder nor with leyt ne with hail ne with pestilence neither
> with war nor with hunger nor wit[h] non other tribulations as
> we have been many times among us for our sins. Wherfore it
> seems well that God loves them and accepts their belief and
> their good deeds.[10]

Mandeville tells of a place where hardship no longer exists,
where plague never ever visits — a paradise beckoning to all
that read. What reader would fail to want a world where he
never hungered and was never ill?

But paradise is not effortlessly maintained even here. God
specifically loves the Bragmanians because, unlike the readers
who have experienced tribulations "many times among us . . .
for our sins," the people of Bragmania "fullefillen the x.
commandementes of God" (211), and are spared. This plague-
free place of Mandeville's creation is not entirely free from
the *threat* of plague. The reader is assured by implication that
sinless behavior has caused the cessation of God's wrath-
ful acts. Were Bragmanians to break the covenant with
God, plague and all other scourges would visit. Readers beware; the Bragmanian model is desirable but difficult to
imitate.

The lesson *Mandeville's Travels* teaches is flawed, finally ineffective, although the story is attractive. Perhaps it inspired hope initially, but it could neither direct nor sustain hope as an action toward an improved end. Too many questions remain unanswered: Who are the Bragmanians exactly? What do they do? How do they worship, or govern, or marry, or raise their children? How is it that they obey all of God's commandments? Mandeville supplies no answer, providing no way for the people of a particular nation to compare themselves to the Bragmanians and thereby learn from them how to banish plague from their nations. Mandeville provides them with a castle in the air: lacking a tether to earth, it is matter of fancy and not of progress.

It would take nearly 150 years before this would change. With the advent of humanism, Italian physicians took the lead, revolutionizing medicine. In England, something equally as original occurred. Utopianism took literary form, growing out of plague-time, and providing the first aesthetic and literary space for praxis in Western Europe. In Thomas More's *Utopia*, the inhabitants control the plague; it does not control them. Plague would not send their leaders into forced exile, because although *Utopia* is fiction, this narrative covers much of the same territory as the plague treatise, another genre growing out of plague-time. In *Utopia*, More tells his readers about Utopian sewage systems, living arrangements, hospitals, health regimens, and medicine. In addition, his Utopians are fully human and know suffering. They inhabit the fallen world shared by More and his readers. They practice solutions to the problems of suffering that all humans share. Readers can follow them, imagining realistically how Utopian solutions might or might not solve England's problems. Thomas More supplied this practical hope in a new literary genre — one emerging in Cantor's "wake of plague."[11]

Many other literary utopias soon followed *Utopia*, among them the little-known 1573 description of Taerg Natrib (Great

Britain). Elizabeth McCutcheon concludes that this description "could be thought of as the first Renaissance utopia to have been written originally in English."[12] More surprising than this little-known work carrying such a distinction are its author and the title of the larger work of which it is a part. The tale of Taerg Natrib occurs within William Bullein's popular plague tale, *A dialogue bothe pleasaunt and pietifull, wherein is a godlie regiment against the feuer pestilence with a consolation and comforte againste death.* A relative of Anne Boleyn, Bullein published medical treatises as well, and toward the end of his career he was a London physician who lived through the violent visitation of 1563–1564. Soon after the visitation, Bullein wrote a dialogue about a group of Londoners who flee from the plague-infected city into the country. Bullein extensively edited subsequent editions, and by the 1573 edition, he had established within his text the link between plague and paradise, between suffering and utopia.

During their flight, Bullein's Londoners meet a traveler named Mendax. This world traveler entertains them for a short time with stories of his adventures, among them an account of the nation of Taerg Natrib and its capital Nodnol (London). The capital, Mendax explains, is strong, lovely, religious, and healthy: "The citie is greate, well walled, and strongly fortified; warlike, with great gates, verie Beautifull, as even Hierusalem was. These gates are locked faste upon the Sabboth, sayving the small portales, to this ende that the Citizens doe not goe, neither ride forth of the Citie durying that dai, excepte it be after the evening praier; then to walk honestlie into the sweete fieldes, and at every gate in the time of service there are warders."[13] During these days of purifying prayer, ministers attend to the young, old, and sick who are left at home. Although the utopian portion of the dialogue is only several pages in length, and most of the attention is placed on Sabbath day worship, it is enough to show readers that in plague-time, the inhabitants of Nodnol practice quarantine, dutifully observe religious prescripts, and care for their physically weak better than those in London do or can.

Within Bullein's plague tale bursts the promise of a "no-place" of improved health. As Mendex concludes his tale, the Londoner proclaims — as the reader may right along with him — "Why, what sight it is, I praie you, or what hearing that is so heavenly" (107). Taerg Natrib is heavenly, but only in the metaphorical sense. It is not Mandeville's nation of pure souls who obey all commandments; walls and warders are necessary not only to keep outsiders out but to keep citizens within. It does not flow with milk and honey, but it does promise that improvements to religious obedience and to health are possible — even in plague-time.

In *The New Atlantis*, Francis Bacon employed the still relatively new genre in an even more extensive manner to prescribe for England's ills. His utopians, the Bensalemites, manufacture odors, tastes, and weather conditions, among many other things. They also enforce a strict quarantine. By these measures, they maintain the sound health of a pure nation: "there is not under the heavens so chaste a nation as this of Bensalem; nor so free from all pollution or foulness," they assert. Untested, untainted, as we would expect from utopia, "It is the virgin of the world"[14] and likely free from plague. Yet even here suffering threatens and demands constant monitoring. Certainly Bacon's visionary mind could have imagined a place of utter peace, as Mandeville had. Like More, however, he chose to infuse his imaginary land with genuine possibility. His utopians, the Bensalemites, are subject to the very laws of nature governing his readers.

The New Atlantis helped to encourage others to follow in pursuit of change. The Royal Society is one of its progeny.[15] In a dedicatory poem for Thomas Sprat's history of the organization, Abraham Cowley helps us understand Bacon's power to inspire utopianism:

>From these and all long Errors of the way
In which our wandring Predecessors went,
And like th'old Hebrews many years did stray
In Desarts but of small extent
Bacon, like Moses, led us forth at last
The barren Wilderness he past,
Did on the very Border stand
Of the blest promis'd Land,
And from the Mountain's Top of his Exalted Wit,
Saw it himself, and shew'd us it.[16]

Like Moses, Bacon is strictly human while also informed and worth following, even into the wilderness. He is the man whose knowledge can help others to the promised land, even though he might never see it. Such a guide to utopia, more specifically, endures suffering that the intended reader can identify as familiar. The guide becomes a trusted ally who shows that a utopia, or any utopian project on a smaller scale, entails suffering as one builds it. One does not simply arrive and relax, as one would in a medieval land of Cockaigne. In their early modern versions of utopia, More and Bacon suggest what Milton will confirm years later: the seeds of plague-time are sown in paradise; humans cannot regain paradise without physical suffering. Once there, they will be required to labor in its maintenance.

An examination of the verb "to suffer" explains the power of the utopian project. From the Latin *sufferer*, "to suffer" means to bear, to undergo, or to endure (OED). Something we bear or endure together is something that can unite us, as in times of grief or during rites of passage. The context might be global, national, local, familial or individual, and the thing we bear might be as mundane as going to the gym or serving for jury duty, but in all cases, the bearing produces a commonality that confirms kinship and promotes empathy among those who endure together. If the reader shares in this suffering, then he or she can imagine that if the utopian society that is so much better has real human beings in it who are "like me," then perhaps the reader's society can follow in some of those new and better measures. Then there is practical hope, a realistic guide to a more prosperous future that begins here and now.

In this context, utopia is not what most of us have assumed: it is not a happy perfect place. It is instead a context in which to illustrate and then animate abstract ideas, seeing whether and to what degree they work, before perhaps employing them in the real world. Modern scholars of utopia, from Ernst Bloch to Lyman Tower Sargent, have clarified the terms: "utopianism" for Lyman Tower Sargent is "social dreaming" and "utopia" is "a nonexistent society described in detail and normally located in time and space" (1).[17] I have adopted these definitions and emphasize the fact that in them, there is no judgment. The new world may be positive or negative or it may be a critique of the utopian project itself. The degree to which the utopia is intended to be better or worse than the contemporary society of the author, or intended as a critique of utopianism in general, will be part of the discussion of future chapters.

Ernst Bloch articulates what I believe is the cause of early modern utopianism and the advent of the genre of utopian literature. Implicit in his understanding of utopia and utopianism is suffering, or a perceived lack of something. The bit that is aching or void, he posits, compels people to wish for something "not yet" that will alleviate their pain or supply what is lacking. The emotion of hope is that drive to imagine and then create or find that which is lacking. For Bloch, hope is the essence of utopianism. In his mellifluous — if not also sometimes meditatively longwinded — three-volume work *The Principle of Hope,* Bloch considers this progression from suffering to a hopeful longing for change and finally to action.[18] He sees each step as a part of real hope and as requiring utopian thinking. With respect to the first part of the progression, from perceived lack to hopeful imagining, Bloch explains that as the sick man "dreams of the body which knows how to keep comfortably quiet again" (2:454), so too the man in whose life "something important is missing" finds that "the dream does not stop inserting itself into the gaps" (1:29). When it grows out of utopian thinking, the dream is a sign of hope that "makes people broad instead of confining them," because "[t]he work of this emotion requires people who throw themselves actively into what is becoming, to which they themselves belong" (1:3). Just as Francis Bacon bore the cause of science in a world not yet fully embracing it, for example, so he becomes an apt model for the newer pioneers of science during the mid-seventeenth century, who likewise faced obstacles set by more traditional peers and patrons. With respect to the content of literary works, Thomas More's narrator Raphael Hythloday plays the same role by laboring even in the telling of what he witnessed in Utopia. He is a model of one willing to throw himself into what is becoming. By witnessing, Hythloday opens the door to utopia for those who hear his story.

From the beginning of the literary utopia, when Thomas More coined the term, to the present, we have been able to distinguish utopia from fantasy by just these means. Utopia always includes some threat of suffering and labor within it, because the hope that founds and then maintains utopia grows out of an awareness that something is lacking or the threat that something will be lacking if action is not taken. Utopia is a world with which the reader can identify, imagining himself or herself within it, trying it on for size. The elements within the literary utopia are those that — like plague — constitute the world of the reader. The difference is that the author imagines them in a different configuration.

The more interesting questions for this study emerge here. What are the limits of hope for a better world in plague-time? To what extent did the best practices prescribed for plague prevention increase or decrease the limits of hope? If the presence of suffering in utopia is necessary, how much is too much?[19] What happens when the utopian dream is shown false, based on what Bloch calls "fraudulent hope": "one of the greatest malefactors, even enervators, of the human race" (1.5)? And to what extent does the study of plague-time literature shed new light on early modern England and her peoples' understanding of and dreams for themselves?

Each of the works in this study provides an intentionally literary and English answer to these questions. To this end, the works here are all products of England, produced by men and women living in an island nation that was clearly distinguished from other nations by geography, climate, population size, religion, and form of government.[20] But first and foremost, these works cohere as literary in their appeal. They are not primarily religious, political, social or ethical prescriptions. They are not at base commentaries on the interpretation of history or on the perceived political power of the authors or of their narrators.[21] As literary works, Thomas More's *Utopia* (1516), William Shakespeare's *Timon of Athens* (1604–1611),[22] Ben Jonson's *The Alchemist* (1610), Francis Bacon's *The New Atlantis* (1627), Margaret Cavendish's *The Blazing World* (1666), and John Milton's *Paradise Lost* (1667) were intended first to capture the imagination of the reader. In the process, the reader embarks on a flight of fancy for the very purpose of recreation, without which one could no better reason than survive the plague. Fancy provided relief, acting as a method by which one could improve the balance of body and mind.

Only after the reader willingly follows does the author of each text reveal his or her more subtle purpose, when one exists at all. And even when there appears to be a purpose at hand other than to supply pleasure, the authors leave their readers to draw conclusions of their own. If there is persuasion, its first form in these works is of an aesthetic nature, entrancing the reader as he or she follows the narrator further and further into the plot. In comparison with the decidedly political utopian literature of the period, which includes Harrington's *The Commonwealth of Oceana* (1656) and Gerrard Winstanley's *The Law of Freedom in a Platform* (1652), the works in this study are aesthetically superior because, among other reasons, they were intended first to entertain.[23]

Moreover, the authors considered here are already familiar to us, already acclaimed for their ability to engage wide audiences, already part of the literary landscape depicted in our courses. Examining their utopian projects side by side and placing them squarely in their plague-time context provides us with a rare opportunity to reconsider our assumptions about these authors and their works. For example, it is a little known fact that before becoming chancellor, Thomas More served two terms as London's Commissioner of the Sewers. His early employment reveals itself in his treatment of infrastructure in *Utopia*, but it may also help us imagine More as a man and not only as a martyr and a saint. In light of seeing his very practical side and of picturing the man toiling over the management of refuse, we come to view More's choices and his writings in a more realistic context.

We can also fruitfully compare authors who are decades and literary worlds apart by viewing their texts as plague productions. For example, we probably would not think at the outset to compare Ben Jonson's *The Alchemist* (1610) and Francis Bacon's *New Atlantis* (1627). Although they appear within two decades of each other, we isolate them by genre. They share much more than a composition date in the first third of the seventeenth century. Each was published within the year after a major plague visitation, each narrative contains the threat of plague, and each has within it a character who, playing the role of the magical *magus*, promises to control nature.

Returning to the questions at hand, it is essential to mark the limits within which men and women could imagine and then work toward a future of improved health. Such is the purpose of chapters 1 and 2. The domain of plague in early modern England begins in physical affliction and in inherited beliefs about the body, nature, and the cause of plague. These factors largely prescribe the paradigm for considering ideal health in the period. When contemplating the paradigm and prescribing treatment from within it, physicians, kings and queens, the clergy, and commoners alike sought the best practices available to them. These practices form the basis for early modern utopian prescriptions.

In chapter 3, I offer a case study. A humanist and a Catholic, who had once been Commissioner of the Sewers and whom King Henry would ultimately select to execute plague orders in Oxford, Thomas More had years of direct experience with and accumulated knowledge of bubonic plague before writing *Utopia*. More knew and employed the best practices of his time. He combined his religious, legal, medical, and experiential knowledge to depict an island on all levels less susceptible to bubonic plague than England had been. The result is a formation of hope peculiar to his culture, on the cusp between medieval and Renaissance.

In chapters 4 and 5, William Shakespeare and Ben Jonson take center stage with a plague-time tragedy, *Timon of Athens* (1604–1611), and a satire, *The Alchemist* (1610). Although each play only very loosely contains a utopian world, each articulates a fear and critique of utopian projects. Written during or soon after visitations of plague that crippled not only the theater but the city as well, *Timon of Athens* and *The Alchemist* contain within them pseudo-utopian worlds from which plague has been banished. Although each play displays a unique picture of the scourge and of the realm intended to repel it, each establishes not freedom from the plague but its very proliferation. The audience is warned: the promise of gold cannot found utopia. Fed by an inability to see beyond immediate needs, promised panaceas will rob men of hope in order to feed despair. Shakespeare and Jonson join the ranks of Joseph Hall and Jonathan Swift, who likewise exposed the potential underside of all utopian projects and of social dreaming in general. In plague-time, they prescribe a healthy dose of skepticism and the wisdom to recognize the fraudulent hope that comes disguised as better places and best practices.

Chapters 6 through 8 treat plague at the advent of the scientific age and return us to a permitted hope, like that in More's *Utopia*. Francis Bacon and Margaret Cavendish wrote numerous and lengthy scientific treatises that include extensive sections on the bubonic plague. Both writers then placed their theories within a utopian literary context — *New Atlantis* (1627) and *The Blazing World* (1666), respectively — and both published their utopian work in volumes containing scientific treatises. Francis Bacon and Margaret Cavendish were in many ways producing like-minded works of scientific and imaginative rigor, each battling the plague with various weapons in an array of arenas. Yet they would not have agreed on the nature of plague or on the purpose and form of utopian literature. Their conception of the relationship between humans and disease was as different as their hope in and prescription for a more prosperous England.

The last chapter, "The Rectification of Air in Plague-Time," revisits the most basic drive to improve one's conditions and the most basic understanding of bubonic plague: it is in the air. John Milton's enormously hopeful energies, directed in plague-time England toward the eradication of sin and the restitution of mankind's original human glory, reveal themselves in his attention to respiration in *Paradise Lost*. We have long known that Milton completed and revised his grand epic *Paradise Lost* during plague-time, when he was self-quarantined in the country during and following the 1666 onslaught. Yet because mention of the literal disease is all but lacking in the poem, scholars have either forced its presence or ignored it, and this has lead to a gap in our account of the poem.[24] A comparison between Milton's Paradise and the city that Margaret Cavendish names Paradise in *The Blazing World* helps to place both works in their cultural context, when air quality received more attention than ever before. Milton and Cavendish clarify the relationship between prosperity and the very literal air by which humans live. Both prescribe increased attention to the power of the air to move individuals and nations toward greater or lesser prosperity. And both showcase plague-time efforts to rectify the air in the hope of strengthening bodies, minds, nations, and in Milton's case, souls.

More, Shakespeare, Jonson, Bacon, Cavendish, and Milton knew humans as flawed and yet deserving of health. They conceived of nations as penetrable and yet well-armed with the best practices. They considered minds prone to fancy and yet sustained by reason. They knew that in a fallen world, societies and the individuals within them would always suffer from internal and external threats. Yet they chose to hope. Employ-ing their sharp minds, visionary imaginations, skill with the English language, and knowledge of the best and most cur-rent practices for improving the conditions of health, they fashioned new answers to old questions. They extended the limits of hope in plague-time.

ONE

Suffering in Plague-Time

The bubonic plague placed many obvious limits on hope in early modern England. Fear of bubonic plague was inherent in all minds from 1348 until well into the eighteenth century. When we review even the most basic facts of the disease as known in an era before antibiotics, we begin to see some of the reasons for its monolithic presence and interpretation. Four out of five people who contracted the disease died within eight days. In the meantime, they developed painful swellings in the lymph nodes as well as scaly, round, red, oozing sores. Any one of these symptoms commanded attention, but the open wounds and buboes elicited the most intense fear. The lymph nodes that tend to swell most are those in the groin area, which is why the swellings are called buboes, from the Greek word for groin.[1]

The suffering brought on by a bubo was not limited to that from the swelling. As J. F. D. Shrewsbury notes, an egg-sized, "hard, painful, hemorrhagic swelling . . . [the bubo is] often palpable on the first day of the disease and is generally conspicuous from the second to the fifth day in the bulk of cases.

If the victim survives this period it may suppurate as a result of secondary infection with phylogenic bacteria and burst on or after the seventh day, discharging much pus and forming a deep ragged ulcer that is slow to heal."[2] No need to exercise poetic license here: even the rather basic description makes us squirm. If the swelling and the stretching of skin were not enough, the bursting should remind us of the movie *Alien*, and this is an apt comparison. It seemed the body was inhabited by a malevolent entity that intended to dominate.

Poets like John Davies did not need to rely on skill to capture the horror of the bubo:

> Now, in his Murdring, he [the plague] observes no meane,
> But tagge and ragge he strikes, and striketh sure.
> He laies it on the skinnes of Yong and Old,
> The mortall markes whereof therin appear:
> Here, swells a Botch, as hie as hide can hold.
>
> (223)

One can imagine the pain when the "hide" has stretched to its breaking point over the botch (bubo): no wonder "some ranne as mad (or with wine over-shot) / From house to house, when botches on them ranne" (241).[3] The explanation of this one symptom accounts for the fear experienced whenever a visitation of plague was rumored, impending, or present. It speaks as well for the power of hope that pulled individuals, cities, and nations forward in such times.

In the 1954 World Health Organization publication *Plague*, specialist Robert Pollitzer cites W. J. Simpson's 1905 description of the second most dreadful of plague symptoms. Carbuncles, Simpson explains,

> rapidly increase in size and then rise in the form of blisters with or without umbilication, while the circumference becomes hard, swollen, and inflamed. The blisters contain at first a clear, serous fluid, which is later dark, sero-sanguinolent or haemorrhagic; and in the contents are plague bacilli. The

blisters soon break and show at their base a moist, bluish-red, inflamed and angry-looking circular or irregular patch, which at this stage may dry up and go no further, or the inflammation may extend to the subcutaneaous tissue, causing a circumscribed or diffuse swelling, the centre of which begins in a few hours to necrose, forming a leathery-looking scab. From this centre the necrosis spreads rapidly to the periphery. The result is the formation of indolent ulcers . . . with hard and red overhanging margins. (Pollitzer, 425)

Although Simpson's standard scientific description of the carbuncle lacks intentional poetic embellishment, it nevertheless captures a sense of intent on the part of the "angry-looking" sore.

Known as "tokens of plague," because they looked like red coins on the body, carbuncles contributed to the popular name for the disease: the spotted plague. A London waterman who became known as John Taylor the Water Poet (1580–1654) captured the commoner's view of these marks in "The Feareful Summer":

Some with Gods Markes, or tokens doe espie
Those Marks or Tokens, shew them they must die
Some with their Carbuncles, and sores new burst,
Are fed with hope they have escap'd the worst.[4]

For a person to survive, it was believed that the carbuncles and buboes must first rupture — hardly a reward for recovery and always unattractive and unsavory.

The famous French physician Ambrose Paré (1510–1590), who served the French monarchy and whose works were well known in England during his lifetime, leaves this account of a house call:

When as I upon a time being called to visit one that lay sick of the plague, came too neare and heedlessly to him, and presently by a sudden casting off the cloathes, laid him bare, that so I might the better view a *Bubo* that hee had in his right groine, and two Carbuncles that were on his belly, then presently a thick, filthy and putride vapour arising from the broken abscesse of the Carbuncle, as out of a raked puddle, ascended by my nostrils to my braine, whereupon I fainted and fell down senselesse upon the ground.[5]

Even an experienced and well-respected court physician such as Paré might topple at the sight and smell of plague. Clearly, it afflicted many more than it killed. Entire households, cities, and nations seemed to swoon, falling into states of ineffectiveness if not coma in its wake.

Many other symptoms accompanied the most famous buboes and carbuncles: malaise, headache, giddiness, apathy or restlessness, nausea, pains in the limbs or lumbar region, inflamed tonsils, and chills due to an extremely high temperature (up to 104 degrees Fahrenheit) within 3 to 24 hours. In addition, the face became flushed and bloated, while hot and dry. The victim had little or no appetite, felt thirsty, and found the tongue so swollen that it might be impossible to keep inside the mouth. The tongue might also appear covered with a pasty white coating, before becoming dry and shiny and then yellowish brownish or even black.[6]

Paré confirms these lesser symptoms: "It is a most deadly signe in the Pestilence, to have a continuall and burning Feaver, to have the tongue dry, rough, and black, to breathe with difficulty, and to draw in a great quantity of breath, but breathe out little; to talk idely; to have phrensie and madness together, with unquenchable thirst . . . daily vomits of greene, blacke and bloudy coulour; and the face pale, blacke, of a horrid and cruell aspect, bedewed with a cold sweat" (833). The plague marked its victims by various yet unmistakable signs regardless of time period or place. For these reasons, people who experienced and wrote about the bubonic plague confirmed that it, and not sweating sickness or smallpox, earned the title the Great Mortality.[7] It was the Great Mortality that pushed people, cities, and nations toward insanity, chaos, and ruin.

The list of symptoms continues, although prolonging the description here would only serve to deplete the spirit and potentially distract us from scholarly examination. Playwright and pamphleteer Thomas Dekker (1572–1632) agreed, changing pace in his own lengthy description of the pest. Clothing the atrocities in dramatic fashion, he provides his audience with a slight respite from the more literal account:

> My spirit growes faint with rowing in this Stygian Ferry, it can no longer endure the transportation of soules in this dolefull manner: let us therefore shift a point of our Compasse, and (since there is no remedie, but that we must still be tost up and downe in this *Mare mortuum,*) hoist up all our sailes, and on the merry winges of a lustier winde seek to arrive on some prosperous shoare.
>
> Imagine then that all this while, Death (like a Spanish Leagar, or rather like stalking *Tamberlaine*) hath pitcht his tents, (being nothing but a heape of winding sheetes tackt together) in the sinfully-polluted Suburbes: the Plague is Muster-maister and Marshall of the field: Burning Feavers, Boyles, Blains, and Carbuncles, the Leaders, Lieutenants, Serients, and Corporalls. . . . Feare and Trembling (the two Catch-polles of Death) arrest every one: No parley will be graunted, no composition stood upon, But the Allarum is strucke up, the *Toxin* ringes out for life, and no voice heard but *Tue, Tue, Kill, Kill.*[8]

Even clothed in caricature, the merciless, horrible onslaught by the "Marshall of the field" and his "Leaders, Lieutenants, Sergeants, and Corporalls" makes clear the warrant for fear.

The physical symptoms of plague were not its only weapons of war. The plague had for centuries practiced terror tactics of surprise, keeping itself well hidden until it had already seized its first victim. By then, it would be too late for many to flee. And it visited like a tornado, leveling one family over its neighbor, one parish over another just a dozen miles away. It was impossible to predict its visitation weeks out.[9] People did what they could and sought signs of plague's more immediate approach.

Most of Europe was familiar with "certain signs" of plague, which were accumulated over the centuries and shared. The signs recorded in Bullein's first edition of *A dialogue bothe pleasaunte and pietifull wherein is a goodly regimente against the feuer pestilence* (1564), for example, are typical, and they include,

> eclipses of the Sunne and Moone, . . . or muche Southe Wind or East winde in the Canicular daies with stormes and cloudes, and verie colde nightes, and extreame hotte daies, and muche chaunge of weather in little time, or when birdes do forsake their egges, flies or thinges bredying under the ground, doe flie high by swarmes into the ayre, or death of fishe or cattell, or any dearth goyng before, these are the sygnes of the Pestilence, and evident presages of the same.[10]

John Davies adds, "No Cat, Dog, Rat, Hog, Mouse, or Vermine vile / But usher'd Death, where ere themselves did go" (230); and Paré notes, "They affirme, when the Plague is at hand, that Mushromes grow in greater abundance out of the earth, and upon the surface thereof many a kindes of poysonous *insects* creepe in great numbers. . . . And also wild beasts tyred with the vaporous malignity of their Dennes and Caves in the earth, forsake them" (821). If a person detected any one or a combination of these many signs, then plague was imminent. Yet, it is hard to imagine that a person would find much comfort in a set of signs so varied and difficult to measure. One sees more mice and more flies out, and this warrants action? It is hard enough for us now to mobilize in the face of a threat, even when we have technology assisting us.

What we do know is that each of these seemingly disparate indicators revealed to them a disturbance in the air. Air could pick up and carry with it noxious fumes from a number of sources. A bog, butcher's heap of leftover carcasses, or open grave might emit vapors and cause all animals and insects in the area to "creep in great numbers" out of their usual habitations. The majority of certain signs indicated what we now call the "miasma theory" of the plague, the most widely accepted theory of the plague's origin at the time. Although the first cause of plague might be God's judgment, he would deliver his punishment according to the laws of nature. He would deliver his deathblow by the air.

Beginning in 1348, the history of plague literature bears out this preoccupation with air and the extensive list of signs by which one might predict a visitation. In that notorious year, the bubonic plague first visited England on its grand tour of Asia Minor, North Africa, the European Continent, The Channel Islands, Iceland, and Greenland.[11] It has been estimated that the mortality reached as high as 50 percent worldwide. Some historians think 20 percent a more accurate number, but that still leaves a grand total of over ten million deaths. In England between 1348 and 1349 alone, bubonic plague killed at least one-third of the population. That fraction does not account for the 20 to 40 percent of people who, on average and regardless of time or place, catch bubonic plague and recover; nor does it take the burdensome and prolonged recovery into consideration. London's loss of population in the same years was worse: one out of two Londoners died.[12]

The impact of this fourteenth century pandemic was at the time heightened by its novelty. Men and women could turn to their priests who might share an apt biblical passage, but there were no plague stories, no national fasts or prayers, no standard plague orders, no colleges of physicians, no bills of mortality — not one national guide for survival, let alone eradication. Rosemary Horrox's collection *The Black Death* shows that within that first year of 1348–1349, a huge European literary corpus developed in response to plague.[13] This corpus remains largely unstudied, and even Horrox's collection is incomplete. From 1348 and well into the eighteenth century, the record of suffering grew.

It is tempting to pinpoint within this plague-time the years of greatest affliction. It is tempting to think that if plague struck more forcefully one year over another that those who wrote about plague in particular years would somehow have a closer proximity to despair and hope or even to the more literal witnessing of physical and national calamity. Using parish records and written testimony from the time, we can assess the number of plague deaths in a given year with some accuracy. But for this study — and, I would argue, for all literary and biographical examinations of bubonic plague — if we first turn to the words of those who lived through the visitations instead of trying to number the dead, we are closer to the experience.

With respect to mortality rates, for example, the Great Plague of London 1665–1666 was by no means the most devastating for the entire country; yet, the writings of Defoe and Pepys make that visitation seem like the only significant plague event in England after 1348.[14] Due to the popularity of Defoe and Pepys among scholars, few people now know that 1593, 1603, 1610, 1625, and 1636 were as deadly, depending upon the parish. No doubt the people of Stratford-upon-Avon considered the plague of 1563–1564 that killed more than 25 percent of their population the "great plague." We might too, knowing that Shakespeare was born during April of 1564.[15] Bristol's civic annals eloquently reveal the relativity of these terms:

> 1544–1545. This year there was a *great plague* in this city which endured for a year.
>
> 1551–1552. This year was the *greatest mortality by pestilence* in Bristol that any man know . . . whereof many people died.
>
> 1565. This year there was a *great plague* in Bristol. The number that died . . . was 2,070.
>
> 1575. This year began the plague to be very hot about St. James's tide, and . . . there died about 2,000 persons.
>
> 1603. In this year . . . began the *greatest plague that ever was* in Bristol . . . and died the number of 3,000 and more.[16]

Every plague-year from 1544 to 1603 was "great" in the minds of those who witnessed and recorded it. The pamphlet "The

Four Great Years of the Plague" provides a visual illustration of the perception (see figure 3).

How, then, can numbers or the descriptions that accompany them put a face on plague or on its victims — those who were literally afflicted and those who watched loved ones die? They cannot. They can point to a larger experience of plague recorded in much broader measure than mortality rates reveal. After all, those outbreaks took place during the years within which the most prominent writers in early modern Europe were born, lived, wrote, and died. Many fashioned guides to plague-time, some forging new genres out of old or adding to tales by their own deaths.

Giovanni Boccaccio's (1313–1375) father died of plague in 1348, as did Petrarch's (1304–1374) Laura, and their writings testify to their experiences. William Langland (fl. 1360–1387) railed against plague-time physicians in *Piers Plowman*. Chaucer's *Pardoner's Tale* (1400) takes place in plague-time, unlike the other previous accounts of the same story. Swiss reformer Huldreich Zwingli (1484–1531) wrote the poem *Plague Song* after his brother's death from plague and after his own successful battle to recover. Erasmus (1469–1536) wrote many letters on his being nearly imprisoned at Oxford while plague raged in London. Hans Holbein, who painted the famous portraits of Henry VIII and Sir Thomas More, died of plague in 1543. Martin Luther (1483–1546) and John Calvin (1509–1564) addressed theological issues attached to flight from the plague. Michel de Montaigne (1533–1592) discussed plague and its effects upon the poor. Edmund Spenser (1552–1599) drew on plague as a setting for his "*Prosopopoia* or Mother Hubbard's Tale." Alvares a Quadra, the Spanish Ambassadour in England under Elizabeth I died of plague in 1563. Jean Bodin (1530–1596), the French natural and political philosopher famous for advocating religious tolerance, died of plague, and it is assumed that dramatist John Fletcher (1579–1625) did as well. Ben Jonson (1572–1637) lost a son to the plague and

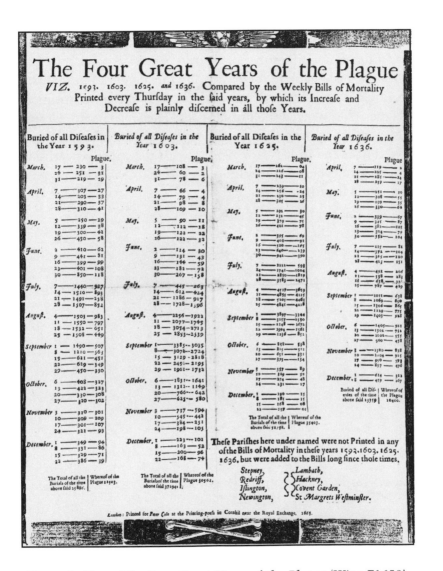

Figure 3. From *The Four Great Years of the Plague* (Wing F1658).
By permission of the Bodleian Library, University of Oxford.

immortalized him in poetry.[17] The list is much longer, and it was not until after 1720, with the last great plague in Marseilles, that the litany would wane.

By the time plague became endemic in England, an extensive and international history of literary, medical, and religious response had begun to take form. By the advent of humanism in England, men and women knew well the proportions of plague. They obeyed the limits it set. They also practiced utopianism, imagining that in the future their children would live longer and in less fear. Those with the most powerful of imaginations began the work of building toward that place of improved health.

Two

The Best Practices
for Change

Those compelled by a vision of utopia to build a bridge from plague-time suffering to a place of improved health began by determining the tools best suited to the purpose. They sought out the best practices available. But before we can identify these plague-time practices, it is useful to determine the platforms on which they were constructed. Any plan to move beyond present suffering and into a healthier future must be built upon preexisting structures. What I call "platforms" are the existing and identifiable frameworks for understanding and modifying the world around us. Religion, technology, economics, science, architecture, and law are some of the platforms on which we build our best practices. These platforms vary by culture. For example, currently in the United States and Canada, technology and economics are the largest platforms. Some would argue that they are largest because they are the strongest, the most likely to sustain future development and to get us from here to there. In another nation, the largest platform might be religion. The individuals in such a nation might conclude that this platform provides the soundest foundation for building an improved future.

Just as we can easily identify the largest of the platforms on which we currently build, we can name those most practiced upon in early modern England, from the time of Thomas More through that of John Milton and Margaret Cavendish, and even to Daniel Defoe. Examining government proclamations and utopian literature together reveals them: religion, natural philosophy (including medicine and regulations pertaining to infrastructure), crowd control (including practices of quarantine and burial prescribed in plague orders), education, and government structure. To improve the nation in plague-time, kings, queens, and those practicing utopianism relied most heavily on the first three of these platforms, and these are my concern in this chapter.[1]

Putting their social dreaming into words, More, Bacon, Shakespeare, Jonson, Cavendish, and Milton built upon each platform to varying degrees. They imagined what the best practices of each platform would look like in the hands of a population who either utilized them more consistently or improved upon them. Before examining each utopian narrative, the place where England's best practices were tested, it is important to reassemble in fuller form the platforms upon which they built those practices.

Religion

In partnership with the medical practitioners and with the government, the church did as much to prevent the plague as was possible from their platform. At government request, the church conducted weekly fasts, printed special prayer books for shut-in families, added plague-specific sermons to all parish services, closed the doors of the church during plague-time, and mandated clergy visits to shut-ins. But each of these practices was, finally, impotent, and the scores of dead clergy made this only too clear.[2] At the same time, the church knew that flight from infected regions was a common practice advocated by doctors and utilized successfully by kings, queens, doctors, and even church officials to escape death. But the church could not advocate flight. The result was a debate without conclusion and a sign that the religious platform could not sustain utopian practices under such conditions. By the time Thomas More was writing, flight had been practiced for nearly 150 years. It seemed to work, but no one could determine whether God wanted people to remain within a plague-infested city and have faith in his protection or whether God wanted people to care for their bodies and families by fleeing from the infection. The Church of England's answer was always the same, as Bishop John Hooper, writing and preaching in 1563, makes clear:

> Although Galen, of all remedies, saith, "To fly the air that is infected is best;" yet I know that Moses by the word of God saith: "Flee whither thou wilt, in case thou take with thee the contempt of God and breech of his commandment, God shall find thee out." Yea, and although many medicines be devised, and assureth the infected to be made while; yet, notwithstanding, I know God's word saith the contrary, that he will send unto unsensible, careless, and willful sinners such a plague and incurable a pestilence, that he shall not be delivered, but die and perish by it. Therefore, forasmuch as sin is the occasion chiefly of pestilence, let every man eschew and avoid it both speedily and penitently; and then shall ye be preserved from the plague sufficiently.[3]

Additional church attendance and fasting were mandatory and those who fled were abandoning their duties to family, church, nation, and queen.

The literary companions for these claims are abundant and often intensified by pitting the city against the country. Those who fled from the city were not welcome in the country, and this divided the nation. In William Bullein's *A dialogue bothe pleasaunte and pietifull wherein is a goodly regimente against the feuer pestilence* (1564), for example, the main character *Civis* flees with his wife from London and into the country. Death follows him, proclaiming, "I will smite thee with this Pestilente darte, as I have doen to many Kingdomes, cities, and people" (177). Flight only brings death faster on one's heels.

Decades later, authors were still complaining that plague caused sinful enmity between city and country folks. The titles alone tell the story: *The fearefull summer, or, Londons calamity, the countries courtesy, and both their misery,* (John Taylor, 1625); *A Looking-glasse for city and countrey vvherein is to be seene many fearfull examples in the time of this grieuous visitation, with an admonition to our Londoners flying from the city, and a perswasion [to the?] country to be more pitifull to such as come for succor amongst them* (1630); *A dialogue betuuixt a cittizen, and a poore countrey man and his wife, in the countrey, where the citizen remaineth now in this time of sicknesse written by him in the countrey, who sent the coppy to a friend in London; being both pitifull and pleasant* (Thomas Brewer, 1636); and *Londons lamentation, or, A fit admonishment for city and countrey wherein is described certaine causes of this affliction and visitation of the plague, yeare 1641.*[4] In each, the country is chastised for its poor treatment of the Londoners in need of charity, and the Londoners who flee are warned that they will find greater charity in London and greater health through prayer.

Very few suggested that Londoners and those in the country might get along. Among them, Brewer's dialogue suggests that on the rare occasion a "Cittizen" might be able to find safe lodging in the country. In order to procure it, however, he first faces rejection, as when the "Countrey-man" initially refuses him lodging, saying simply,

> Why sir, whence come you? Masse [I] feared you
> From London, where the Plague is parlous hote,

And it be so, no further words but mumme:
No meate, nor drinke, nor lodging will be got.

(A2)

We can imagine that upon seeing the citizen dressed in his city attire, the countryman plugs his nose — the sign employed in most literary treatments of the city versus country. The first page of Brewer's dialogue includes an illustration of this very gesture (see figure 4). The end of this tale is unusually positive, however, because the wife of the countryman comes along and discovers that the citizen is a Christian. At this, the countryman and wife decide to open their home and have a feast to show their good charity, and no one dies. Much more typically, these narratives end in the death of all involved; in such cases — as depicted in the image from the 1641 pamphlet *Londons lamentation. Or, A fit admonishment for City and Countrey* — people from the city are better off remaining within the more charitable city than fleeing to the cruel country (see figure 5).

In the abstract, all agreed that if one remained in London during visitations, this indicated great faith and goodwill, and that if a Londoner came into the country looking for lodging, the Christian thing to do would be to open one's home to him. Of course, we must assume that people generally enforced these practices only in the abstract; they became the stuff of poetry and prose precisely because they rarely occurred. People fled and those in the country treated them cruelly. Each action spoke less of charity than of a desire to save one's own skin, and neither spoke of faith in God. The church had little room for interpretation, and its general policy on flight would not change.

The matter was even more complicated when it came to members of the clergy and their own safety in plague-time. The people might be encouraged, when not ordered by the Privy Council, to avoid church congregations in plague-time, but the *Book of Common Prayer* decreed that the preacher must visit his afflicted parishioners at home if necessary.[5] At the same time, it was well known that with earlier plagues more clergy died than laypersons. This issue was hardly a small matter; it drew the judgments and soul-searching of the most prominent religious authorities of the time.

By 1603, the issue of flight became more contentious. Angered that the official plague orders in England had for decades prescribed only medical remedies and crowd control, Henoch Clapham and others believed the nation needed a warning. In *An epistle discoursing vpon the present pestilence* (1603), he exhorts,

> Beloved, God having smitten our Citie with the Pestilence, Behold, booke upon booke, prescribing naturall meanes as for naturall maladies, but little said of spirituall meanes, for spirituall maladies, which should give liefe to the former. To speake and act in such cases, as sole Naturians, is of Christians to become *Galenists*, and of spirituall to become carnall. If a true Christian do but take meate or drinke, hee prayeth for a blessing: because otherwise *the dead creature can give to him no life*, nor yet continue health. The tru Christian taketh no Phisicke for the weakest ague or ache, but hee calleth upon the name of the Lord for adding his blessing; for that otherwise the thing applied, can remove no maladie. For the true Christian hath learned, not only to *Pray continuall, and in all things to give thankes*: but also that *Every creature of God is good*, being *sanctified by the word and Prayer*.[6]

By refusing to admit the necessity of natural remedies and precautions, Clapham challenged, the king, doctors and those clergymen who had fled from plague or who had somehow made their peace with the decree of crowd control and medical regimen.

The official and printed plague orders had warned,

> If there be any person ecclesiasticall or Laye, that shall hold and publish any opinions (as in some places report is made) that it is a vain thing to forbeare to resort to the Infected, or

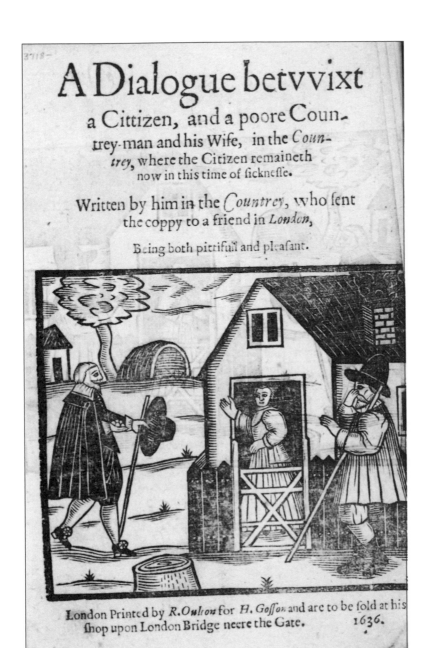

A Dialogue betvvixt

a Cittizen, and a poore Countrey-man and his Wife, in the *Countrey*, where the Citizen remaineth
now in this time of sicknesse.

Written by him in the *Countrey*, who sent
the coppy to a friend in *London*,

Being both pittifull and pleasant.

London Printed by *R. Oulton* for *H. Gosson* and are to be sold at his
shop upon London Bridge neere the Gate. 1636.

Figure 4. From Thomas Brewer, *A Dialogue* . . . (STC 3717.5).
Title page. By permission of the Huntington Library.

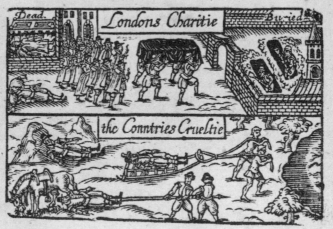

LONDONS LAMENTATION.

Or a fit admonifhment for City and Countrey,

Wherein is defcribed certaine caufes of this affliction and vifitation of the Plague, yeare 1641. which the Lord hath been pleaf:d to inflict upon us, and withall what meanes muft be ufed to the Lord, to gaine his mercy and favor, with an excellent fpirituall medicine to be ufed for the prefervative both of Body and Soule.

Londons Charitie

Dead.   Buried

the Conntries Crueltie

London, Printed by E. P. for Iohn Wright Junior. 1641.

Figure 5. From *Londons Lamentation* (Wing L2934). Title page.
By permission of the British Library.

that it is not charitable to forbid the same, pretending that no person shall die but at their time prefixed, such persons shall be not only reprehended, but by order of the Bishop, if they bee Ecclesiasticall, shall be forbidden to preach, and being Lay, shall be also enjoyned to forbeare to utter such dangerous opinions upon paine of imprisonment, which shall be executed, if they shall persevere in that errour.[7]

Clapham acted alone and was never punished. And although he was a Calvinist and not in a position of power within the Church of England, he expressed the opinion of many who found the plague orders sorely lacking in spiritual prescription. Later, Puritans would take up similar claims and challenge traditional Galenic medicine and the government that supported it by adopting Paracelsian medicine. The division would reach its height by the 1630s.

By 1603, however, we see the lines drawn as clergymen in the Church of England attempted to reconcile plague orders with church teaching. Lancelot Andrewes, the famous Bishop of Winchester who would help give shape to the King James Bible and whom Milton would celebrate in elegy, was among those who attempted to capture the reconciliation in words. He responded to Clapham directly. In *Doctor Andros his Prosopopeia*, Andrewes explains that one cannot with good conscience dismiss the natural causes of plague:

Myne opinion is that how soever there is no mortality, but by and from a Supernaturall cause, so yet, it is not without concurrence of naturall causes also, for the most parte. And that as the former by fastinge and prayer and such like spirituall meanes to be removed; so the latter may and ought to be avoided by naturall courses and meanes. And I clearlie and expresslie hold the plague to be infectious and that it is most expedient for the parties infected, to be severed and shut up (thy having things necessarie and convenient provided for them) expedient also for the sound to forbeare the companie of such as are infect; as also a lawfull and honest meane to escape the receaving of

like contagion. That a faithful Christian man, whither mag-
istrate or minister, may in such tymes hide or withdrawe himself, as well corporeally as spirituall, and use local flight to a
more healthfull place (taking sufficient order for the discharge
of his function). Besides, that neither all that escape at such
tymes have faith; nr that all that [ ] want it.[8]

In this statement, Andrewes reinterprets the best practices
advocated by the church: fasting and prayer. But as fasting
and prayer help the spirit ward off the plague, flight is a natural
course for preserving the body. For Andrewes, the two practices
go hand in hand. There is no need to select one over the other,
and in fact one would be foolish to do so. In plague-time,
Andrewes advocated utilizing the best practices of religion in
concert with those of natural philosophy and crowd control.

But Andrewes is unusual in expressing such opinions
publicly, and Clapham would not let the dispute rest. In 1605,
he published Andrewes's response and then added his rebuttal
point for point. Clapham argued that although there might
seem to be two causes for plague, natural and supernatural,
there were actually two separate forms of plague. Flight might
prevent the natural plague, but "flight prevents not the supernaturall stroke" (29). In fact, by failing to trust in God and
fleeing from the natural stroke, one might sin and receive the
supernatural plague as just punishment. Moreover, although
catching the natural plague and even dying from it would not
automatically condemn your soul to hell, failing to trust in
God could deliver the double blow of physical death combined
with an eternity of pain for the soul in Hell. Andrewes did not
respond again. The decision of whether to flee or stay would
play in the minds of men and women well into the eighteenth
century, where it became the primary point of contention in
Daniel Defoe's *Journal of the Plague Year*.[9]

Regardless of the official policies, clergy members did more
often flee than remain at their posts. In such cases, they left
their parishioners with an astonishingly well-developed set

of resources that were slightly more concordant with those prescribed by doctors than one might gather from the preceding focus on flight. Clergymen could not advocate flight, but they could, for example, adopt the language of the medical practitioner and even acknowledge the value of Galenism in other areas. In a letter preceding his 1563 homily, Bishop Hooper wrote to all pastors and curates in the diocese of Worcester and Gloucester to explain just this relationship between the plague-time prescriptions of the church and those of Galenic medicine:

> I have thought it my bounden duty, seeing at all times I cannot comfort the sick myself, to collect or gather into some short sermon or homily a medicine and most present help for all men against the plague of pestilence. . . . And whereas Galen saith that *"Omnis pestilentia fit a putredine aeris;"* that is to say "All pestilence cometh by the corruption of the air, that both beast and man, drawing their breaths in the air corrupt, draweth the corruptions thereof into themselves" he saith well, yet not enough. He saith also, very naturally, that "when the air is altered for from his natural equality and temperature to too much and intemperate heat and moisture, pestilence is like to reign." . . . Yet that is not enough. As Ezekiel saith, where as God sendeth all these distemperances, and yet Noah, Daniel, and Job were in the midst of them, they shall be safe. (160–61)

Hooper adds to a Galenic diagnosis without denying its credibility. He reminds his parishioners that God is the first cause. As long as they remember this, they are free to attend to the air.

The conversation was not one-way. Early modern doctors were likewise positing the final cause of the plague as within God's will. Often the doctors' final conclusions echoed the preachers'. For example, within his first chapter of *A Treatise of the Plague*, entitled "The causes and cures of the Plague," Thomas Lodge asks his readers to turn to the Bible for explanation:

> This Sickness of the Plague is commonly engendred of an infection of the Aire, altered with a venemous vapour, dispearsed and sowed in the same, by the attraction and participation whereof, this dangerous and deadly infirmitie is produced and planted in us, which Almightie God as the rodde of his rigor and justice, and for the amendment of our sinnes sendeth down upon us, as it is written in Leviticus the 26. Chapter, and in Deuteronomy the 28. *If you observe not my Commaundements saith our Lord, I will extinguish you by the Plague which shall consume you.*[10]

It is telling that a physician of high repute such as Lodge cites *Leviticus* 26 and *Deuteronomy* 28, neither of which has to do with the healing of the physical body. Instead, through these passages and his unmistakable use of them, he asserts that the cause and potential increase of plague directly results from the breaking of God's commandments.

The church openly and proudly owned the very origin of plague. The clergy did not need to be present for their parishioners to know this. All understood that plague visited when God deemed it necessary. Yet while the church might be said to own the origin of plague, it could never own or even imagine its cure. In more concrete terms, the debate over flight indicated that the church would never be able to build into their arsenal of best practices against the plague a practical, real-world prophylaxis to the extent that doing so would save lives. The church's platform could not support the best practices for building a future of improved health. In early modern English utopian literature, the Church of England would have to appear in quite altered form — when it appeared at all.

Natural Philosophy

Natural philosophy supplied the platform from which early modern men and women understood their relationship to the natural world. What makes up the air we breath, our bodies, and our minds? How do we differ from animals? What causes death? Natural philosophy supplied answers through medicine and advocated practices for improving air, bodies, nature, and minds. Providing support for the entire platform was Galenic theory. By the time Thomas More wrote *Utopia*, doctors had spent nearly 150 years failing to cure the disease. Still, most practitioners of natural philosophy remained true to Galenic doctrine and practice.

Given the very slow pace of change in early modern medicine compared to the rapid developments in our own time, paradigm shifts with respect to thinking about plague within the period are generally easy to mark. The first shift occurred with the discovery of Galen's original Greek texts. Prior to this, practitioners worked with Arabic translations of Galen. With the originals, they could gain ground on Galen, approaching more directly what they believed was the truth in his teachings. This first shift occurred in Thomas More's time and provided him with access to the best practices available. The second shift would occur over 100 years later with the introduction into England of what has become known as Paracelsianism. Each shift brought change — slow change, from academy to commoner over decades. But the changes appear in utopian literature slightly earlier than in other cultural products, and in order to understand the literary texts, it is essential that we consider first the general trends in natural philosophy that run through them.

Based on a theory of balance among the four humors (black bile, yellow bile, blood, and phlegm), Galenism was the codification of Hippocratic theory, which had trickled down to English practitioners and commoners in various forms over the centuries since its origin. Muslim clerics had translated original texts into Arabic, and these survived for translation into Latin. With the rediscovery of the Greek originals in the early sixteenth century, European practitioners hoped that they could get closer to the true source of medical wisdom, and a translation campaign ensued. European universities that could claim mastery of the original Galenic corpus secured authority. English doctors studying abroad decided England should not be left behind.

Adding to the growing interest in an old master, the newly discovered original texts emphasized flexibility in the practice of medicine. Each patient was different. Each prescription must be suited to the individual.[11] Thomas Linacre, a close friend of Thomas More, was one of the men who determined that England would not be left behind. He soon succeeded in convincing Henry VII to build new hospitals in England and to support the creation of the Royal College of Physicians, in which all members had to study and practice Galenic medicine. Doctors in plague-time England would have the most advanced understanding of bubonic plague available in the western world.

Through the lens of Galenic medicine, the picture of bubonic plague is quite different from the ones we currently view[12] — a disease with a discrete set of symptoms and a single origin. But Galenic medicine instead interpreted every physical and psychological ailment as a symptom of bodily imbalance, not as the result of a particular agent. A host of symptoms presenting together might constitute a disease, but each symptom would be treated separately.

More specifically, Galen viewed each human body as composed of seven "naturals": among them, elements, qualities, *spiritus,* and the now-famous four humors, which we best understand. Affecting the naturals were external conditions known as "non-naturals," including air, exercise, food, drink, sleep, coitus, and affections of the mind. Too much or too little of any of these, they believed, would bring about a change in the naturals. The naturals would become imbalanced and produce "contra-naturals," aptly named. Contranaturals included pus, vomit, fever and other violent efforts made by the body to return to its original condition of balance.

This very reasoning led Galen to the following diagnosis of plague, based on what we now call the miasma theory. Any vaporous, heavy, or otherwise seemingly tainted air (non-natural) could invade the body (composed of the naturals). If the air was not fit for respiration, the spiritus and then the body as a system would overheat. In the normal process of digestion, the stomach essentially cooked food into the right amounts of bodily fluids or humors for balance. Too much heat or too little and the body converted food into an imbalanced mess of fluids. In an effort to restore balance, the body would try to expel the excess, which by this time would have putre-fied into contranaturals. In the case of an extremely noxious inhalation, the result might be such an overproduction and putrefaction of humors that the body had no choice but to push them out in the form of buboes, carbuncles, and fever, and other obvious symptoms of plague.[13] In such cases, nature seemed absolutely unnatural as the body fought against itself, risking its own external wounding for the sake of internal balance.

It was simply a matter of adding sin and God's wrath to the Galenic model, and one could Christianize the chain of events in the following way: excessive, sinful passion leads to God's wrath. God then sends a noxious vapor, a non-natural intended to disturb human bodies passing through it. The introduction of the vapors into the already sinfully imbalanced body would cause excessive imbalance, and plague was born, fiercely decked out in buboes and carbuncles. This Christianized Galenic understanding of plague was firmly established by More's time. It was the only way to understand disease as it functioned in the natural world.

We find this Christianized Galenism throughout popular literature of the time, from ballad to play to prose pamphlet.

For example, Bullein recalls the trouble plague brings to those who attempt to flee from the pest. The Medicus in *A dialogue bothe pleasaunte and pietifull* recites to his patient, "The Pestilential fever, saieth Hipocrates, is in twoo partes considered: the first is common to every manne, by the corruption of the air. The second is private, or particular to some men, through evill diete, repletion, which bryngeth putrifaction, and finally, mortification. And Galen in the differences of fevers, doeth affirm the same" (49). Bullein's knowledge of Galenism, distributed here in a popular form, is highly accurate with respect to its source, and he follows with an exhaustive list of some of the many causes of plague:

> Privies, filthie houses, gutter, chanilles, uncleane kept: also the people sicke, goyng abrode with the plague sore running, stinking and infecting the whole, or unwise rashe passing with an emptie stomake out of the house: Neither to sitte tippling and drinking all the daie long, nor use running wrestling, Daunsyng, or immoderate labour, whiche dooe not onely open the pores but also cause the winde to bee shorte, and the pulses to quick, and the arters drawe to the harte when it panteth, the pestilenciall ayre and poison. And what is worse then fear of mind, when one doeth heare ill tydyng, the death of the father, mother, child, &c. By it the spirites and blood are drawen inwards to the harte. Also of care, anger wrath &c. These are al perilous. (62)

"Care, anger, wrath" and fear "when one doeth hear ill tydyng" are each non-naturals that, when introduced to the body, can disrupt the naturals and make one more susceptible to plague. To counter this, Bullein concludes in step with Galen: "mirth must be used specially in this case" (62).

Mirth is a hallmark of Galenic treatment, and a crucial prescription, key in the understanding of literature at the time; yet, it is easily eclipsed in studies by the methods of phlebotomy, which are so much more gruesome. Like the letting of blood, mirth was thought to maintain balance of the humors.[14] But how was one to practice mirth in such dark times? In *The Wonderfull Yeare* (1603), Thomas Dekker points out how very difficult it is to practice mirth or even seek consolation in plague-time, because the very things that bring us mirth shift: "How many upon sight only of a Letter (sent from *London*) have started back, and durst have laid their salvation upon it, that the plague might be folded in that emptie paper, believing verily, that the arme of Omnipotence could never reach them, unlesse it were with some weapon drawne out of the infected Citie" (59). Even letters from loved ones might drive one to fear, making one more susceptible. If they brought good news and caused mirth, however, letters might instead fortify one against the plague. Like a letter bomb, one would not know until it was too late.[15]

Galenic medicine seems to be entirely inadequate to us now, but it did lend sufferers, their loved ones, and practitioners some peace of mind. It suggested that there was a degree of causality: one might witness a chain of events in the natural world and determine the right steps to take to prevent harm. Thomas Lodge is one of the many physicians who put his faith in this Galenic reasoning. The subtitle of his *Treatise of the Plague* (1603) proclaims this confidence: *A Treatise of the Plague: Containing the nature, signes, and accidents of the same, with certaine and absolute cure of the Fevers, Botches, and Carbuncles that raigne in these times: And above all things most singular Experiments and preservatives in the same, gathered by the observation of divers worthy Travailers, and selected out of the writings of the best learned Phisitians in this age.*[16] A "certaine and absolute cure" of plague symptoms is possible, because Lodge follows "the writings of the best learned Phisitians in this age." In fact, Lodge only considers physicians learned only if they utilize the theories Galen and Hippocrates. He mentions the two early authorities on nearly every other page in spite of his claims that in the end, prayer is the more reliable healer.

Always accompanying the potential comfort supplied by the Galenic physician, however, was pain. Because it was believed that buboes must rupture and heal prior to any chance of recovery from plague, for example, the Galenic physician would help the process along by cupping and lancing. Ambrose Paré paints a vivid picture:

> So soon as the Bubo appears, apply a Cupping-glasse with a great flame unto it, unlesse it be that kinde of Bubo which will suddenly have all the accidents of burning and swelling in the highest nature; but first the skinne must be anointed with the oyle of lilies, that so it being made more loose, the Cupping-glass may draw the stronger and more powerfully; it ought to sticke to the part for the space of a quarter of an houre, & be renewed and applied again every three quarters of an houre, for so at length the venom shall be the better and sooner bee absolved and perfected. (853)

Following his directions, Paré records the attempts of victims to heal themselves: "There are many that for feare of death, have with their owne hands pulled away the *Bubo* with a paire of Smithes Pincers; others have digged the flesh round about it, and so gotten it wholly out. And to conclude others have become so mad, that they have thrust an hot iron into it with their owne hand, that the venome might have a passage forth" (854). Atrocious or not, this account suggests just how powerful the Galenic prescriptions had become.

With respect to pain, the victim of plague was likely better off if attended by family than by doctors. Those taken to a pest house were worst off. The first plague houses functioned essentially as death houses, far enough removed from the city that the sick could not contaminate the living. As F. P. Wilson reports, they were never intended to aid the afflicted: "Most of the patients were houseless, moneyless, or friendless people who regarded the pest house with horror. Its management, like that of the prisons, was farmed out to keepers who were often extortionate in their charges and harsh in their treatment" (68). The plague house stood as prevention for the healthy and persecution for the dying.

Very few people ever made it to the plague house to begin with. There simply were not enough of them. In 1516, Thomas More had written in *Utopia* that any well-governed city had pest houses. He wrote because London did not have one. It did not 68 years later when Queen Elizabeth declared that the city needed one within the walls to keep the ill cordoned off from the healthy. Ten years after this, we find Thomas Nashe comparing London to cities in other nations that have several plague houses: one for those not yet showing signs of plague but likely infected, one for those infected with unburst buboes, and one for those with ruptured sores who are on the road to recovery.[17] Only in 1594 was a pest house constructed in London. Yet this facility was soon determined inadequate.

The average person relied on a vast oral tradition of healing, which included herbal remedies and parts of the Galenic, which corpus had trickled down to the masses. Codification of this oral tradition took the form of regimen books that delineated full programs of health. Sir Thomas Elyot, knight and author of the popular *The Booke Named the Governor* (1531), for example, wrote his own regimen. Entitled *The castel of helthe gathered, and made by Syr Thomas Elyot knight, out of the chief authors of phisyke; whereby euery man may knowe the state of his owne body, the preseruation of helthe, and how to instruct well his phisition in sicknes, that he be not deceyued,* Elyot's book went through over a dozen printings, from 1534 to 1610 — more reprints than *The Booke Named the Governor.*

Elyot's regimen is typical in its emphasis on moderation in all things. In a short section at the end entitled "A diete preservative in the tyme of pestilence," he explains,

The bodies most apte to be infected, are specially sanguine, next colerike, than fleumatike laste melancolyke, for in them the humour being colde and drie, is most unapt to receive putrifaction, having also strayte passages, by which venim must passe. The diete convenient for the tyme is to abstein from metes, inflaming and opening the pores also from the heat of the sonne, from to moch heate of fire, or garmentis, from very hot herbes, and moche use of tart thinges, except onions and cikory, or radishe with vineger. For they do resist against venim. . . . Beware of lechery, of a clowdy wether and close, eshewe moche resorte or throng of people, wyndes commynge from fennes or mores, from slepe at none. . . . In the mornynge, at a temperate tyme kembe your heed backward, clense your body and heed of all superfluities: use also moderate fricasies, with swete perfumes, and odours, washe oftentimes your face and handes with pure vyneger myxt with rosewater.[18]

Elyot continues to list foods and hygienic practices that will preserve one against the pestilence. In doing so, he clearly adheres to Galenic causality: an imbalance in the naturals (heat, moisture, etc.) or in the non-naturals (air, food, sleep, emotion) brings about plague. Regulation of the non-naturals will help restore balance.

Elyot also highlights some of the prominent Galenic themes and images that we can trace in literature during this period: purging of undesired elements from a system (heart, mind, body, city, nation), and fear of things that might create an imbalance in the humors (passion, anger, greed, but also travel, exile, sex, falling into a cave or being kept in a dungeon or smelling a potion). A Galenic "no place" that was safe from plague would be a place where the air was clear, emotions were temperate, and the citizens regulated their habits in every area of life. In the next chapter, we will see this very utopia: dating from roughly the same period in English history, it will come complete with Galenic themes and images.

Yet, as securely embedded in the culture as Galenic medicine was, the pestilence brought it into question. The general theory of the humors would persist for decades after the plague's last visit, but the lack of efficacy opened the door to new ways of viewing the world and the body's relation to it. Particularly appealing to imaginations were the new chemical treatments attributed to Paracelsus (1493–1541). In general terms, those prescribing chemical remedies were prescribing what they believed to be the essence or the spirit of a mineral distilled through processes known to us as alchemical. To apply this thinking to plague diagnosis and remedy, it is helpful to consider Paracelsus's general theory of disease.

The son of a Swiss physician, Paracelsus came into the world with the name Theophrastus Phillippus Aureolus Bombastus von Hohenheim. It seems he also came into the world to question it. Early in his life, he came to the conclusion that Galenic medicine he had learned through men like his father had failed to include God and astrology in the very composition of human bodies and minerals. To rectify the situation, Paracelsus coined the name by which we know him and traveled through Europe spreading a theory based on Platonic correspondence between microcosmic and macrocosmic bodies. In the process, he would make many enemies, but he would also open many minds to new ways of thinking about the interrelatedness of God, nature, and humans.

Paracelsus's ideas did not catch on immediately, because they were an extreme departure from Galenic medicine, and because Paracelsus believed more in active practice than in codification of knowledge in books. He wrote very little, but it takes only a short description of his paradigm to understand why few initially listened to him. Paracelsus considered all created entities, from human beings to planets to minerals, as consisting of both secular and sacred parts. Each body had within it a sacred "astrum" that acted as the informing principle of the secular body. We might call this astrum a soul or a virtue: metaphorically, if the astrum is a stamp, it gives form and function to the wax, which is the body. Paracelsus also believed that the astrum of one body could impress its stamp on another by any number of means. Paracelsus considered diseases to have their own autonomous astrums as well.

In this way of thinking, disease was an individual agent capable of producing symptoms. In *From Paracelsus to Van Helmont,* Walter Pagel sums up this contrast between Paracelsian understanding of disease as an entity in its own right and the Galenic conception of disease as a general imbalance in the humors made manifest by a host of symptoms, which as they varied signaled different diseases: "In other words," Pagel says, "what varies [in the Paracelsian view of disease] is not the subject (the patient), but the object (the disease)."[19] Galen's remedies were herbals and surgery directed not at the disease but at the patient's humoral imbalance as revealed by symptoms. Whether fever, ache, or boil, symptoms indicated a humoral imbalance and not a specific type of disease. Symptoms, then, could only reveal imbalance. Simple, yes, but Paracelsus saw Galenic medicine as flawed from the outset. Paracelsus would insist that physicians should learn to understand the origin of each individual disease rather than wasting time on the back end, fiddling with minor symptoms of humoral imbalance. And he believed it took a *magus* to peer into the origin of each disease. Only a wise and spiritual man could discern the correspondence between the astrum of a particular disease and the astrum of a mineral that could provide perfect remedy for the diseased astrum of the human body. Within the Paracelsian paradigm, the cause of bubonic plague looked quite different than it did to the Galenic practitioner. For Paracelsus and others prescribing chemical remedies, the body's astrum was imprinted with an evil astrum, ultimately as a punishment for sin. No vapors or humors were involved. One ill seed entered one body. For treatment, one chemical distillation — sometimes the combination of a number of minerals — replaced cupping, lancing, and purging.

In literature, we can see these differences in themes related to prophecy, astrology, the power of the magus, the coming of the golden age made by man's new relationship to nature, the need for a revolution, and an emphasis on travel over book-learning.[20] A Paracelsian utopia would entail more radical change, and Paracelsian utopians would emerge as little gods and as heroes after a successful revolution. They would look like Shakespeare's Prospero and dress like Jonson's Subtle, or like one of the fathers in Bacon's Temple of Solomon. Galenic utopians, on the other hand, would have evolved slowly through the adoption of sound habits. They would have mastered quite naturally regimens such as those prescribed by men like Sir Thomas Elyot, and they would look quite a lot like More's Utopians.

But we find only glimpses of Paracelsianism in English texts by the beginning of the seventeenth century. It challenged Galenism as a theory but never came to close to changing the way most people thought about and prescribed for their bodies. One of the reasons for this is that Puritans came to champion the Paracelsian cause for largely political rather than medical reasons, and this force kept Paracelsianism in a marginal position. When we see Paracelsianism in literature, it is often displayed overtly but embodied in one character or posited as a single contending theory among many. In contrast, the Galenic influence in literature can almost escape our notice, because it is everywhere sewn in. It was likely taken for granted even by the authors employing it, just as we may use Freudian terms like "projection" and "repressed" without intending to signal their origin in our readers' minds.

For all of their differences, Galenic and Paracelsian medicine share the notion that disease is inherent in the human condition. Galen could not have imagined the elimination of imbalance in the humors any more than Paracelsus could have posited an utter cleansing of sin or an end to minerals, the nonspiritual waste expelled by the earth in its own process of digestion. Often the two branches of medicine came together in plague-time for another reason: when the disease was plague, medical authority became the sufferer. No cure cured. No preventive medicine succeeded. Thomas Dekker noted in *The Wonderfull Yeare* (1603),

> Never let any man aske me what became of our Physicians in this Massacre. . . . I cannot blame them, for their Phlebotomies, Losinges, and Electuaries, with their Diacatholicaons, Dia-codions, Amulets, and Antidotes, had not so much strength to hold life and soul together, as a pot of Pinder Ale and a Nutmeg: their drugs turned to durt, their simples were simple things: Galen could do no more good than Sir Giles Goosecap: Hippocrates, Avicen, Paracelsus, Rasis, Fernelius, with all their succeeding rabble of Doctors and Water-casters, were at their wits end, or I think rather at the worlds end, for not one of them durst peepe abroad. (36–37)

Hippocrates fares no better here than Paracelsus.

The inadequacies of medicine were noticed on all levels of Elizabethan and Jacobean society and abroad, as John Davies of Hereford notes,

> All observ'd the Pestilence was such
> As laught to scorne the help of Phisickes art;
> So that to death All yeelded with a touch,
> And sought no help, but help, with ease to part.

> (229)

To many it seemed that doctors had constructed the best practices for bringing pain rather than for securing improved health.

On the other hand, there were many who put their support of practitioners into writing. For example, after venting his anger at ill-prescribing doctors, John Taylor makes certain to remind his readers that

> This sharpe invective no way seemes to touch
> The learn'd *Physitian*, whome I honour much,
> The *Paracelsians* and the *Galennists*

The Philosophicall grave *Herbalists:*
These I admire and reverence, for in those
God doth dame *Natures* secrets fast enclose
Which they distribute as occasions serve
Health to reserve, and health decai'd conserve.

(A10–A11)

Not everyone despised doctors — or at least not all of the time. Some, as above, had faith in them.

Others admired doctors, as surgeon William Clowes explained in 1602,

> Much strife I know there is between the Galenistes and the Paracelsians, as was in times past betweene Ajax and Ulisses, for Achilles armour. Notwithstanding, for my part, I will heere set up my rest & contentation, howsoever impertinent and unseemely soever it make shew. That is to say, if I find (eyther by reason or experience) any thing that may be to the good of the Patients, and better increase of my knowledge & skill in the Arte of Chirurgery be it eyther in Galen or Paracelsus; yea, Turke, Jewe, or any other Infidell: I will not refuse it, but be thankefull to God for the same.[21]

Many doctors did all they could in the face of incurable disease and certain pain, and by their persistence, they led the way for others to believe that something better was just around the corner. More, Bacon, and Cavendish placed this other side of the corner squarely within a utopia that both controlled for plague and kept doctors on call. The presence of plague and of doctors takes different forms in each text, but all of them reveal the degree to which early modern English men and women put faith in the best practices of natural philosophy.

Crowd Control

The monarchy put its faith in crowd control. To avoid the spread of plague, they terminated all large social gatherings. They ordered the closing of ports, postponed Parliament, relocated their entire court when threatened, restricted travel, and supported stricter building policies to prevent crowding. They controlled the population as well as we do today. Yet, with all of these best practices from which to select, they learned only the hard way and over time how to plan ahead, to act offensively rather than defensively. It takes but a brief look at the erratic plague-time course charted by Henry VIII to realize that sometimes the best practice for the king was not always the best practice for the nation.

If we read the itineraries of Henry VII, Henry VIII, Edward VI, Elizabeth I, James I, and Charles I in this way, they become a series of plague-escaping movements rather than royal progresses. Henry VIII's reign in particular was a record of running matched by none. In "The Progresses of Henry VIII, 1509–1529," Neil Samman charts Henry's early travels and concludes, "Disease, or rather Henry's fear of disease, was one of the biggest influences upon the court's itinerary and the progress. In most years it was the plague which affected the court. . . . In less dramatic years the plague still continued to shape the king's itinerary to a lesser or greater extent and only [the itineraries of] 1516 and 1519 appear relatively unaffected by the threat of disease" (71). Henry's fear of disease left the entire court at the mercy of the plague, as was well known by all who surrounded him.

Made more extreme because of his desire to live to produce an heir, the king's fear grew out of consistent near-encounters. In response, Henry acted as if he were waging a series of battles — in the each case, yielding the field to plague in order to save his neck.[22] In the first year of his rule there was a severe outbreak in the garrison of Calais, as well as great plague in diverse parts of England. Two years later in July of 1512, Elizabeth Woodville, mother of Edward V and Henry's grand-mother, died from plague. The ambassador of Venice had written that Henry — 21 at the time and just three years into his reign — had become clearly anxious over that death.[23] A few years later, in March of 1518, Henry was still encountering plague not only within his kingdom but also within his household. Three of his pages died of the disease while he was in Richmond. Again he was forced to flee, as Creighton explains,

> On the 6th April it was decided by the king's privy council at Abingdon that London was still infected and must be avoided, the queen (Catharine of Arragon [sic]) having declared the day before that she had perfect knowledge of the sickness being in London, and that she feared for the king, although she was no prophet. On the 7th April the report of four or five deaths at Nottingham ("as appears by a bill enclosed") was made the ground of postponing a projected visit of the king to the north. (290–91)

Flight after flight, Henry and his court encountered the plague.

In 1520, attempting to keep well away from the plague's domain, Henry purchased Hunson Manor in Hertfordshire "specifically as a country retreat from the plague."[24] This measure worked, but plague would strike much closer to home, when in 1532 the master of the kitchen died from plague, only one day after having waited upon Henry.[25] This was also the year in which it was rumored that Anne Boleyn had caught the plague and survived. We do know that only four years later, and soon after Henry VIII had Anne executed, he was married and still fleeing from plague. He postponed the coronation of Jane Seymour, "seeing how the plague reigned in Westminster, even in the Abbey."[26]

By October of 1537, he had even more reason to restrict access to his royal family. Jane Seymour had produced Henry's male heir. Yet due to his fear of the plague, the king had not been with mother and child at the birth. He chose to remain in Esher while she delivered Edward in Hampton Court.[27] Later, Henry celebrated in London, where, according to historian W. K. Jordan, "the bells were rung, 2000 salvos were fired from the Tower and a high mass was sung at St. Paul's, while ale and wine flowed in the streets for all to take. Plans were at once drawn, in which the king played an active role, for the christening of the infant on the third day after birth."[28] The original proclamation that accompanied the announcement of the birth, however, tells a different story. Plague had again altered the king's plans:

> Forasmuch as it hath pleased Almighty God of his infinite goodness to send unto the King our most dread sovereign lord a noble prince to the great comfort and welth of this realm . . . his highness, being credibly informed that there is and hath been great infection of the plague within the city of London and the suburbs of the same, doubting that a great multitude of his loving subjects being joyous (as they have cause) of the birth of the said noble prince would make their access to his grace's court, whereby peril might ensue, doth therefore straightly charge and command all and singular subjects, of what estate, degree, or condition soever he or they be, that they nor any of them shall repair or resort unto his said grace's court upon Monday next but only such as be appointed by his special letters from his highness or some of his council . . . upon pain of the offenders of this his grace's proclamation to incur into his majesty's most high indignation and displeasure.[29]

At least Henry's lineage was secure — as any, that is, in plague-time. He would care as best he could for Edward, declaring that none of his household was to visit London or any other place in the summer months when there was danger of plague. Any sick person in the household was to be withdrawn at once.

But at what cost to the nation did Henry VIII secure his own head and his lineage? The plague kept him on the run, and as Thomas More and Cardinal Wolsey knew, this left the nation dependent upon messengers who would convey royal decrees by horse across the nation. When our heads of state leave on vacation, even now we feel that the nation is slightly unmanned. Still, we rest assured that telephones, the Internet, and other technological advances keep our presidents in control. We rely on those best practices to keep the country running and to see us safely into the future. Early modern England's kings and queens instead threw themselves into patterns of flight, in essence throwing themselves at the mercy of plague and leaving London vacant for occupancy.

This was no way to secure the prosperity of a nation, but such was the inherited and seemingly best practice for avoiding plague. And indeed, no king or queen in plague-time ever caught the plague. It would appear that the plague-time practices Henry VIII had inherited from his father worked. Henry VIII passed this particular inheritance on to his own children who likewise fled in times of visitation. By the time Edward VI and Mary came to the throne, flight as a reason for initiating or altering the royal progress had become accepted and was regularly initiated for all sorts of reasons, making it less disruptive.[30] Henry VIII's flights had foreshadowed those of his children, showing them that monarchs should run when plague came knocking on the capital door. By flight, a king or queen could stay only one step ahead of plague. It may in fact have been a method to stay away from rather than ahead of plague, and it certainly left no energy for utopian thinking. What king in flight from an enemy could simultaneously plan for the future? Retreat is not advance. Running away from something is not the same thing as taking steps to neutralize or at least lessen a threat.

While Henry ran, many of his counselors, Thomas More among them, put their energies into the imaginative flight that would produce blueprints for a better nation. Henry's daughter Elizabeth may have been among those practicing utopianism. When it came to protecting herself from plague, she acted more often by decree than those before her. In 1564, for example, she established a gallows in Windsor to hang anyone daring to visit from London. In 1585 she forbade the importing of wine from infected regions, and in 1589 she limited the freedom of soldiers returning from contagious regions in Spain and Portugal.[31]

Most important of all, in 1578, she put into place a set of plague orders that applied to all parishes in the realm. Their title accurately suggests their intended power: *Orders thought meete by her Maiestie, and her privie Councell, to be executed throughout the Counties of this Realme, in such Townes, Uillages, and other places, as are, or may be hereafter infected with the plague, for the stay of further increase of the same. Also, an advise set downe upon her Maiesties expresse commaundement, by the best learned in Physicke within this Realme, contayning sundry good rules and easie medicines, without charge to the meaner sort of people, aswell for the preservation of her good Subjects from the plague before infection, as for the curing and ordring of them after they shalbe infected* (see figure 6).[32] She knew that her father's flights and piecemeal decrees were not suitable. Perhaps this is in part because she had encountered plague in her own home years earlier. In January of 1548, exactly one year after her father's death, the 14-year-old Elizabeth's tutor of three years, William Grindal, died of plague.[33] Elizabeth grew up with the knowledge that plague was deadly and must be shunned. To a larger extent than her father, Elizabeth battled plague proactively through what we might call prophylactic proclamation.

As the best practice for crowd control, nothing else replaced Elizabeth I's orders. In the years following her reign, James I, Charles I, Cromwell, and Charles II would turn far more often to royal proclamation than to progress as they sought to control the plague. The most obvious signs of their direct inheritance of plague prescriptions from Elizabeth are their plague orders, each of which follows almost to the letter that first issued by Elizabeth in 1578.[34] Each of the monarchs drew from a full arsenal of weapons inherited from the previous king or queen. Elizabeth I made the most comprehensive strides. She

ORDERS,

thought meete by her

Maieſtie, and her priuie Councell, to be
executed throughout the Counties of this Realme,
in ſuch Townes, Uillages, and other places, as are, oʒ
may be hereafter infected with the plague, foʒ
the ſtay of further increaſe of the ſame.

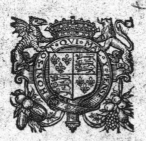

⟐ Alſo, an aduiſe ſet downe vpon her
Maieſties expreſſe commaundement, by the beſt learned in Phyſicke within this Realme, contayning ſundʒy good
rules and eaſie medicines, without charge to the meaner
ſoʒt of people, aſwell foʒ the pʒeſeruation of her good
Subiects from the plague befoʒe infection,
as foʒ the curing and oʒdʒing of them
after they ſhalbe infected.

⟐ Imprinted at London by Chriſto-
pher Barker, Printer to the Queenes
moſt excellent Maieſtie.

Figure 6. From Elizabeth I, *Orders, thought meete by her Maiestie*
(STC 9187.10). Title page. By permission of the Huntington Library.

insulated herself and her court, as if she were an island within an island, and at the same time, she prescribed for the health of her people. In this way, her policies and actions approximate those of More's land of utopia and Bacon's Bensalem, where visitors face security checks at the border so that inhabitants can live with limited threat from disease.

THREE

Thomas More's Pestilence in Parentheses

By the time Erasmus quarantined himself in 1513, people were wearied by the pest and knew well what precautions to take. Like Erasmus, who sequestered himself in his quarters at Cambridge University, they knew to confine themselves in regions unaffected by plague. They waited. And like Erasmus, they were hopeful for improvement: "The plague is raging as fiercely in London as the war is with you," he wrote to his friend, the king's Latin secretary Andreas Ammonio. "I am therefore staying at Cambridge, looking every day for a convenient moment to take wing, but no opportunity occurs."[1] A month later in early October of 1513, Erasmus wrote to William Gonnell: "Things here are just as before; so I am thus far undecided whether I ought to return to join you. Once again there has been a death not far from the college, and Bont the physician has died, out in the country, as has his little daughter at home. Therefore please oblige me by not changing the beds for four days. If I come, I shall come with our friend Watson" (2:255). Erasmus had returned from a visit with Gonnell in the country and, although it was safer there, he feared venturing out while plague was at his doorstep. Still, he remained watchful, ready to flee to better conditions.

The coming months would see Erasmus in flight from Cambridge to London and into the country and back again, always writing to friends and colleagues about his hope for healthier times and sustained companionship. During these months, he may have thought about how accurately he had rendered the subject of plague-time friendship in *Oration in Praise of the Art of Medicine* (1499):

> How much more genuine a friend is the physician, he who after the fashion of the birds of Seleucis (which, they say, are never seen except when their protection is neede against a plague of locusts destroying their crops), never intrudes himself upon those who are hale and hearty. But in times of peril, in these adversities in which wife and children often abandon a man, such as in cases of phthiriasis, consumption, or pestilence, the physician alone is constant in his attendance, and he is present, unlike many others, not out of mere sense of duty, ineffective as that is, but is there to give practical help, is there to contend with the disease for the life of the critically ill, and thereby frequently puts his own life at risk.[2]

The best friend risks his life in order to give comfort. Erasmus's particularly strong affection for his English friends only increased the pain of separation, and his letter to John Colet in 1506 confirms this: "There is no land on earth which, even over its whole extent, has brought me so many friends, or such true, scholarly, helpful, and distinguished ones, graced by every kind of good quality, as the single city of London. . . . I cannot but be sharply hurt by the pangs of separation from friends such as these."[3] Plague-time demanded extended separation from those on whom one relied, those from whom one might normally seek solace in hardship. In some sense, plague turned Erasmus's friendships against him.

Thomas More was one of Erasmus's close friends in England. The years Erasmus spent in almost constant self-quarantine are those leading up to the publication of More's *Utopia* in 1516. They are also the years during which Thomas More had accepted governmental positions that demanded attention to issues of social health in London. By 1511, Thomas More was appointed undersheriff of London. Although the records of his duties are meager, it is certain that in this capacity he provided legal advice to the sheriff during court proceedings regarding the city.[4] Whenever the king ordered enforcement of a new policy, More would advise the sheriff of his legal obligations and of the methods by which the sheriff might best uphold the decree. A large number of these decrees revolved around the health of the city. More's duties necessarily extended to interpreting sanitation policy and seeing that it be put into practice.

One area of general concern in London was the notoriously poor quality of the water and air. Butchers leaving fleshy filth in the streets to fester and dumping it into the Thames contributed to the problem. The deposited flesh would rot, smell, and cause general discomfort, concern, and potential illness — seeming to taint the air with foulness. In a Galenic understanding of disease, vapors from rotting flesh and other refuse transmuted the air and disturbed the "naturals" of those who inhaled it. Without proper sewage systems and methods for clearing garbage, London was for decades a ripe environment for plague and a big headache for those in charge of sanitation.

Ernest L. Sabine's venerable study "Butchering in Medieval London" confirms that during plague-time, people grew increasingly concerned with the general dumping of waste in their waterways and streets.[5] As early as 1391, when plague again visited London, her inhabitants protested against the butchery practices. One hundred years later, by the time More was a young boy, complaints had not diminished. By 1511, when Thomas More was undersheriff, it was clear that larger health and sanitation reform was imperative. Four years later and a year before the voyage to Antwerp, which would see him begin *Utopia*, More was appointed as Commissioner of the Sewers. With this post came an even more direct role in keeping the streets and waterways of London cleared of plague-causing filth.[6] With this post and that of undersheriff came the extra burden of knowing exactly how and why one's friends were hemmed in by plague. With this post also came knowledge of crowd and sanitation control.

In the years after More wrote *Utopia*, he would renew his role as Commissioner of the Sewers and take even larger steps to secure the nation from plague. In January 1518, More was selected to enforce the very first royal plague orders issued in England. His particular assignment took him to Oxford in April. The king had recently fled from plague in London and was residing in Woodstock, half a dozen miles from Oxford. He and the court were anxious. They feared the plague would find them. Only one month earlier, three pages in the court had died of the disease. Someone needed to secure Oxford, someone trustworthy, knowledgeable about plague, and just expendable enough. The king could better afford the loss of an essential member of court than a risk to his own life. Thomas More succeeded in his assignment, reporting from Oxford what was by English standards at the time good news: only three children had died, and all houses where the pestilence was or might soon be visiting were clearly marked. With Oxford thus secured — its contagious citizens identified and isolated and its dead at a minimum — the king could breath more freely, passing by if necessary.[7]

But well before More's occupation called him to confront the plague, he had learned through firsthand witness that "its hard with Subjects when the Sovereigne / Hath no place free from plagues, his head to hide."[8] Erasmus was not the only one who proclaimed a fear of plague and whose actions were often curtailed by it. He was not the only one who hoped for the no place — an *ou-topos* — that was free from plague. Thomas More knew that bubonic plague was virulent in 1500, as Henry VII flew from infected Calais. A year later, More had witnessed Catharine of Aragon's first meeting with her intended Prince Arthur. The original rendezvous had been postponed, leaving Catharine on the ship and away from Gravesend's plague-ridden port. Thomas More had written of viewing Catharine upon her final arrival there: "Everyone is singing her praises. There is nothing wanting in her that the most beautiful girl should have."[9] More's attention and loyalty were secured from that moment on, and he would have heard of her brush with death.[10]

By 1502, More was in his second year in residence with the Carthusians at the London Charterhouse.[11] Plague raged about him there in London and nearby at Oxford and Exeter, where, according to Charles Creighton, "two mayors died of it in quick succession and two bailiffs" (289). More might have felt safe within this Carthusian monastery, because it was well fortified against the plague — well fortified with prayer. It had in fact emerged out of a plague visitation. When the Black Death visited London in 1348, it came with such force that men, women, and children were dying without secured burial space: too many corpses, too few graveyards. In the hope of remedying the dismal situation, three different men with three different charitable donations and intentions bought plots of land just outside London's city walls. All three plots were consecrated as graveyards.[12] Just over a dozen years later, in 1361, the Bishop of London died from the plague. He had been one of the three original founders of the cemetery and was buried along with thousands of plague victims. His connection to the land was made even more permanent by his will, which paid for the foundation of the London Charterhouse upon the grounds. In this way, he established a chantry where the monks in residence would continuously pray for the souls of those buried nearby. The Charterhouse, where More wrote his speech on Augustine's *City of God* and where he contemplated a life of monastic service, paradoxically owed its existence to the bubonic plague.

Surrounded by tombs, the Charterhouse residents would have known their duty: constant prayer for the souls of plague-victims, so that those souls might one day escape the pains of Purgatory. The monument in the Charterhouse churchyard reminded everyone within of this purpose:

> *Anno Domini* 1349. *regnante magna pestilentia, consecratum fuit hoc Caemiterium, in quo & infra septa presentis monas-terii, sepulta fuerunt morturorum corpora plusquam quin-quaginta millia, praeter alia multa abhinc usque ad presens, quorum animabus propietur deus Amen.*

> Anno Domini 1349, while the great pestilence was reigning, this cemetery was consecrated wherein, and within the walls of the present monastery were buried more than fifty thousand bodies of the dead, besides many more from that time to the present, on whose souls, may God have mercy. Amen.[13]

In such a setting where once *"regnanate magna pestilentia,"* Thomas More and the Carthusian monks could little doubt the power of plague over individual lives and entire popula-tions. As devout, pre-Reformation Catholics they would not have questioned the necessity of their prayers in the saving of souls. This was their calling. By the time Thomas More wrote *Utopia,* he had a working understanding of the best religious practices for plague prevention and healing: prayer unceasing.

More's understanding of the plague was as complete as possible for the time. He knew the best practices of crowd control and of religion, and as a result of his 11-year friendship with Thomas Linacre, he knew how to build on the platform of natural philosophy.[14] Linacre had acquired medical training in Italy from 1487 to 1497. At the time, Italy was the leading country for medical education and facilities. At the University of Padua alone, where Linacre received his medical degree, there were 35 instructors on the medical faculty in 1467. For an Italian medical school, this was not unusual. In contrast, England did not see formal lectures in medicine until 1550.[15] Linacre's return to England prompted him to establish better medical education and healthcare in the nation. He knew what he needed to do: inspire his prominent friends to support him, create a lectureship at Oxford that would bring in educated practitioners to train English students, and establish a guild for the training and licensing of doctors.

Thomas More was one of his earliest advocates, but Linacre had also gained the attention of the king. By 1504, Henry VII expressed a considerable interest in public health, founding an almshouse at Westminster for the poor and sick. Four years later he expanded his plan to include three other hospitals — all for the sick poor, not just for the healthy poor, as was the norm. The largest of the three hospitals was created in the Savoy Palace building and was chiefly based on the hospital pattern of the Santa Maria Nuova. As Linacre had hoped, it appeared that Italy would lead the way to England's health reform.[16] Linacre and his many patrons, including More, imagined they would one day see England rival Italy; in which case, it would lead the world in medicine.

This would not come to pass. England would not surpass other nations in healthcare. But Thomas More's land of Utopia would. It rivaled all nations by its best practices of medicine. Its citizens would be healthier than England's or any other known population. In all other cases, *Utopia* as a narrative is anything but simple, as we know even from its name. "Utopia" originates with More's creation and is a combination of the Greek words for *eutopos* and *outopos*, "happy-place" and "no-place" respectively. This contradiction in terms is still troublesome, and it has demanded further definition by scholars like Lyman Tower Sargent, whose terms I have adopted. If we follow Sargent's definition for utopia as "a nonexistent society described in considerable detail and normally located in time and space,"[17] then we have a suitable term for More's, because it in no way suggests whether or not More intended his Utopia as a model.

When we return to the text, we see why we need latitude in our discussion. Scholars must grapple with More's very basic presentation of *Utopia*. A story within a story, *Utopia* was written in parts over many months and in two different countries before undergoing editing at the hand of Erasmus and others. The choice of narrator adds to the complexity of the account as well. Thomas More creates a character named Raphael Hythloday; when translated, Hythloday means "talker of nonsense." He is our guide to the island, but with such a name, can we believe any of what he says about his adventures? Are we supposed to laugh at the nonsense? Or is the wisest of men a fool, a talker of such nonsense, as Erasmus suggests in *Praise of Folly?* The scholarly jury continues to ponder these and other points of interpretive tension. But one thing is clear: with respect to health measures, England would be better off if it followed the example of the Utopians.

As Hythloday describes Utopian infrastructure, for example, we glimpse More as Commissioner of the Sewers imagining improved conditions for England: "Outside the city are designated places where all gore and offal may be washed away in running water. From these places they transport the carcasses of animals slaughtered and cleaned by the hands of slaves."[18] Hythloday explains in detail that the Utopians simply, "do not permit to be brought inside the city anything filthy or unclean for fear that the air, tainted by putrefaction, should engender disease" (4:139). The marginal notes contributed by Erasmus confirm the fear, calling the reader's attention to the association of "infectious" air, butcher's filth, and plague: *"Tabes ac sordes pestem inuehit ciuitatibus"* ("Disease and Filth Introduce Plague into the Cities"). Quite clearly, Erasmus's note underscores the relation of decay (*tabes*) and filth (*sordes*) to plague (*pestem*).[19] The Utopians have eliminated this particular cause of plague, and we can be certain that More's readers, like Erasmus, saw the butcher-regulating measures as plague-prevention.

Free from pollution, the water supply for Utopia is also constantly self-cleaning, never standing: the water "passes the city uncontaminated. When the ebb comes, the fresh and pure water extends down almost to the mouth of the river." Then, "in case of hostile attack [when] the water might be cut off and diverted or polluted," they have another river with water "distributed by conduits made of baked clay" (119), a veritable circulation system with pure blood cleansing the entire body. Where the ground does not permit such conduits — as was often the case in London — "the rain water collected in capacious cisterns is just as useful" (119).[20] In order to subsist on rainwater, the Utopians' air must have been free of pestilent vapors. For the air to remain pure, the water — and if we extend this, the sewage system in general — must have been in exceptional order by early modern standards.

More generally, the Utopian's temperate use of all resources — or in one word, their utility — is their best method for maintaining health. Galen would have agreed: the best health is delivered when all of the various parts of the body are working together, functioning neither above nor below their natural levels. All Utopian practices, institutions, and citizens are functional and peaceful because they exist in a well-ordered concord. Their humors are balanced, self-regulated by a regimen that makes them automatically better able to withstand a pestilent vapor than their English counterparts.

All Utopian ideas and institutions reflect this emphasis on utility accompanied by an appreciation of natural variety. We find these very ideas in Galen's *De sanitate tuenda*, one of the works translated by Linacre. The best constitution of a

human body for optimal health is "that which is best pro-
portioned, which has the conformation of its parts best suited
to their functions, and which, in addition, exhibits every
number and size and mutual relation of all parts advantageous
to the actions. According to our standards, the ideal body
weight is midway between thin and corpulent . . . hirsute or
bald, soft or hard."[21] Health is a matter of coming closest to
this condition of balance:

> Since health is a sort of harmony, and since all harmony is
> accomplished and manifested in a two-fold fashion, first in
> coming to perfection and truly being harmony, and second in
> deviating slightly from this absolute perfection; so hygiene
> should also be a twofold harmony, one exact, optimal, abso-
> lute, and perfect; the other deviating slightly from this, but not
> so much as to harm the animal. (13)

Health is a harmony, an always-changing attempt to bring what
is imperfect into line with the ideal.

Assessing the particular relationship between these states
of perfection and imperfection is crucial, for the ratio varies
in each individual: "For neither do all healthy people see
equally with their eyes, but some more and some less; nor do
they hear equally. . . . If, therefore, differences of functions
correspond to differences of nature, it follows that there are as
many differences of nature as difference of function" (13–14).
The best hygienist will know how to determine the individual
natures peculiar to individual people. The Utopians have
likewise learned to accept and even cherish a diversity of
practices that suit them as they differ by age, skill, and desire.
The best health of the state or body must accommodate and
to some degree encourage variety while maintaining a harmony of the individual parts. Because no two individuals
are the same, the best regimen for maintaining health is a
self-regulated one, as Raphael Hythloday records, "Even
though there is scarcely a nation in the whole world that needs
medicine less, yet nowhere is it held in greater honor — and

for this reason that they regard the knowledge of it as one of
the finest and most useful branches of philosophy" (4:183).
Each citizen finds in medicine what they find in gardening:
medicine is *pulcherrimas atque utilissimas* (finest/most beautiful and most useful), just as gardens are described as being to
the citizens both useful (*usum*) and delightful (*voluptatem*).[22]
Each citizen acts as his or her own physician, for each knows
best his or her own nature and the functions displaying it.
When the function changes, the Utopian knows to strive again
for the right individual balance.

There are times in Utopian medicine, unlike in Utopian law,
when an expert is necessary, so Utopians have retained their
medical practitioners, even though very little in their nation
contributes to illness. The lifestyle on all levels is preservative.
When disease visits, it is highly unlikely that Utopians will
fail to diagnose and seek to cure it. It would seem that Utopians
have achieved what Galen considers the optimum of conditions for health. As if he were writing about More's Utopians,
Galen describes the perfect conditions of health:

> Let us now discuss the ideal constitution, of which each part
> has a wholly perfect nature. Such a person, placed under the
> art of hygiene, would be fortunate if entrusted to it immedi-
> ately after birth. For thus he would benefit psychologically,
> since advantageous regime would develop desirable habits. But
> even if he came under hygienic care at some after age, he will
> derive the gretest advantage therefrom. We shall first point out
> how, if one took such a person from the beginning, one would
> keep him healthy through his whole life, unless some external
> violence should befall him, for this does not concern the prac-
> tice of hygiene. (22)

Start the Galenic hygiene at birth and the child will be physically and psychologically sound. The Utopians are reared in
Galenism from birth, not as a regimen one memorizes but as
a lifestyle. In this way they achieve and even exceed Galen's
expectations.

Galen had written that violence upon the human body caused by factors outside of one's control — tempests, pestilence, famine, and so on — "does not concern the practice of hygiene." More's Utopians move one step beyond Galen in having taken preventive measures against even such extremes. For the most part, those preventive measures work. Famine does not exist, war is rare and controlled when it occurs, and tempests do not harm the well-fortified island with its cities nestled in the interior cove. Disease, including the plague, is nearly eliminated. As they guard themselves against war and are prepared with measures to care for their wounded, they are carefully composed for every event with infrastructure and medical knowledge unparalleled in More's lifetime.

Utopian hospitals reveal both More's realistic approach to his new world and his knowledge of best practices. His fictional hospitals would rival those Linacre had seen in Italy. Hythloday provides the details: "special care is first taken of the sick who are looked after in public hospitals. They have four at the city limits, a little outside the walls" (4:139). By the end of the sixteenth century, only two hospitals for the care of the physically sick existed in London, and London had more hospitals than most towns. Utopians, in contrast, had four for each of their 54 cities: 216 public hospitals on their island. Utopia accommodates all sick, and the accommodations are both efficient and comfortable. Each of the 216 hospitals is "so roomy as to be comparable to as many small towns. The purpose is twofold: first, that the sick, however numerous, should not be packed too close together in consequent discomfort and, second, that those who have a contagious disease likely to pass from one to another may be isolated as much as possible from the rest" (4:141). Moreover, "these hospitals are very well furnished and equipped with everything conducive to health. Besides, such tender and careful treatment and such constant attendance of expert physicians are provided that, though no one is sent to them against his will, there is hardly anybody in the whole city who, when suffering from illness, does not prefer to be nursed there rather than at home" (141). The "constant attendance of expert physicians" is given to all equally, regardless of wealth, something of which the English might only dream. Not a single English man, woman, or child no matter how sick would have preferred "to be nursed" in the English hospital "rather than at home."

The problem with managing healthcare in England came largely from the origins of the facilities themselves. Prior to the Renaissance, hospitals were church-sponsored hospitality centers providing room and board to weary pilgrims, supportive patrons, and aged or chronically ill brethren. When an inmate was ill, the first priority was isolation, then comfort. The guiding principle was that the sick person should not interfere with communal obligations.[23] The similarity in floorplans for all monastic infirmaries of the time attests to their primary function: a long rectangular room with beds on either side lengthwise lead to an altar around which most of the daily routine took place.[24] The shape of the hospital was that of a church, and in order to maintain their keep, even the lay patients were required to pray for the souls of the local deceased and living.

When patients did receive treatment for their physical afflictions, it was at the hands of the *infirmarius* whose first responsibility was administrative. There were never doctors on staff, and no medical training was available to the clergy. There may have been a medical textbook available to the *infirmarius*, but some monasteries determined that the *infirmarius* was not allowed to treat illnesses.[25] Only the fortunate ill — if there was such a thing — found themselves under the care of a Shakespearean Friar Lawrence, who knew of herbal remedies and had no fear in prescribing them.

By our standards, healthcare was disastrous in More's time; nevertheless, More understood its value. Rather than eliminate hospitals from his Utopia, for example, he improved them on all levels. Utopian hospitals are large, clean, efficient, well staffed, with special care for those with contagious diseases. Perhaps most novel, Utopian hospitals are "little cities" devoted to the care of sick bodies, while English hospitals were cramped, dirty, disaster zones devoted to care of the soul. This was an enormous advance from what More knew in England. On the platform of natural philosophy in England, he learned the best practices from other humanists like Linacre, and then improved on what he found. By doing so, he created a defense against the plague that none had yet come close to matching.

Reading Hythloday's description of the island, and remembering that More was writing in plague-time, we can only conclude that Utopia would never need fear a visitation. Its air, water, and citizens are self-cleansing and therefore always well humored, while still human and imperfect. Raphael reminds us, for example, "though they have not a very fertile soil or a very wholesome climate, they protect themselves against the atmosphere by temperate living and make up for defects of the land by diligent labor. Consequently, nowhere in the world is there a more plentiful supply of grain and cattle and nowhere are men's bodies more vigorous and subject to fewer diseases" (4:179). By means of a careful regimen on all levels — agricultural, spiritual, social, etc. — Utopians, living in this "nowhere" maintain a high degree of fitness. If Raphael were to tell us that Utopians have never experienced the plague, we might at this point believe him.

He can report no such thing. In an interesting digression on population control, Hythloday explains what happens when Utopians grow too numerous. This is a worthwhile consideration, given that health, exceptional fertility, and longevity lead to exponential population growth. It makes sense that Utopia would become too crowded to maintain quality of life. Unlike dystopian societies we have read about, Utopians do not practice forced birth control, limit the number of children permitted, or have a cutoff date for life, after which citizens are recycled as food. Instead, when the population exceeds a reasonable limit, Utopians send citizens to other nations, where they live in established colonies.

Then Hythloday brings on the surprise. The Utopians have a plan for the opposite scenario:

> If ever any misfortune so diminishes the number in any of their cities that it cannot be made up out of other parts of the island without bringing other cities below their proper strength (this has happened, they say, only twice in all the ages on account of the raging of a fierce pestilence), they are filled up by citizens returning from colonial territory. They would rather that the colonies should perish than that any of the cities of the island should be enfeebled. (4:137)

Plague did visit Utopia, twice wiping out vast numbers of the population.

This one mention of the literal disease in Utopia — in a parenthetical statement within a digression no less — hardly indicates an author's obsession with, or even concern over, a particular health risk. Certainly, More displays an island so well ordered that plague has been all but eliminated. He might have stated more directly and specifically that Utopian health leaves so little room for plague that it has *only* visited twice in their entire history. Twice is next to none when compared to the numerous visitations England had experienced by 1516.

An examination of Thomas More's use of parenthetical statements in *Utopia* helps to clarify the situation. The Latin text must be the basis for such an examination, as translators rarely retain the marks "(" and ")" that open and close the parenthetical statement wherein More mentions *pestilentia*. It is easier for the meaning, most editors assume, to eliminate the marks and turn the subordinated material within them into phrases connected to the main clause by commas. However, this can alter the meaning of the text.

John Lennard accounts for the oversight of translators and scholars when it comes to the employment of "lunulae" or "round brackets" that mark parenthetical statements: "The distinction between the rhetorical figure and the lunulae often used to mark it is crucial, for while the rhetorical figure dates to classical antiquity (Cicero often used it), the practice of marking is not found until 1399, [and] is specifically associated with humanism."[26] The marks became an issue of communication in the age of the press, right about when More was writing *Utopia*. Erasmus was in fact the first person to coin a term for them, calling them "lunulae" because they are shaped like the waning moon.[27] During that time, the printing press was revolutionizing reading, writing, and thinking. One result was a rethinking of punctuation: how can we signal to the reader when to breathe, when to view something as an aside, when to read with greater or lesser emphasis, and how can we do it on the cheap? Printing was costly, so punctuation needed to assist the reader with emphasis and the publisher with economy. Other marks had once signaled the parenthetical statement, but none served as efficiently as the lunulae.

Lennard goes on to explain and demonstrate that contrary to our contemporary definition of the parenthetical statement as an aside or digression unnecessary for complete understanding of the passage, "the new technique was rhetorical, acting on the page to emphasize" (5). The lunulae most regularly indicated *sententiae*, dependent clauses, vocatives, comparisons, attributes of speech, and so on. Humanists expanded this range, taking punctuation quite seriously. They knew that punctuation was one of the few ways to control the audience's reading and perhaps comprehension in the age of the printing press.

Specifically, More's lunulae in *Utopia* function to facilitate the conversational quality of Hythloday's dialogue. Beyond using the lunulae for a "(she proclaimeth)" or for a common proverb, More most frequently employs his first lunula, the first round bracket in the set, to signal that an aside is occurring: the narrator will address the reader as in a soliloquy.[28] By means of the first lunula, Hythloday breaks out of the dialogue to speak directly to the audience who is sometimes the character of More, sometimes the reader, sometimes both. The end of the seeming soliloquy is the second, closing lunula.

Hythloday's first lunulae prove the point. More tells Hythloday that he "would make an excellent member of any king's council," and Hythloday replies, "You are twice mistaken, my dear More. . . . In the first place almost all monarchs prefer to occupy themselves in the pursuits of war — with which I neither have nor desire any acquaintance — rather than in the honorable activities of peace" (4:57). The translator has dropped the lunulae around *"quorum ego neque peritiam habeo, neque desydero"* ("with which I neither have nor desire any acquaintance"). By dropping it, the emphasis of the rhyming "neither . . . nor" in *"neque peritiam habeo, neque desydero"* is lost. We can, nevertheless, imagine Hythloday speaking to More and emphasizing his utter lack of desire for or understanding of the proceedings in princes' courts. The parenthetical statement clarifies Hythloday's position with regard to the subject. It is addressed directly to More and all others in the audience, readers included. When we do not consider the remark as an important aside containing Hythloday's more personal remarks, we learn of Hythloday's dislike for court positions, but his utter rejection of the idea is not emphasized. We have less of the character and less of the story if we misread the lunulae.

The majority of *Utopia*'s lunulae signal just such points of intimate emphasis, as in their very next appearance: "At the time," Hythloday explains to More, Peter Giles, and John Clement, "I was much indebted to the Right Reverend Father, John Cardinal Morton, Archbishop of Canterbury and then also Lord Chancellor of England. He was a man, my dear Peter (for More knows about him and needs no information from me), who deserved respect as much for his prudence and virtue as for his authority" (4:59). Again, Hythloday speaks directly to his audience, both to the character More and to the reader who in More's time had no doubt known of Cardinal Morton. In this case, the translator retains the lunulae, showing how clearly the marks function to signal the direct address of the audience. Hythloday displays familiarity with his audience and with what that audience might need in order to follow his story with ease and interest.[29]

In light of this reading, More's placement of plague within lunulae highlights its occurrence in Utopia. Within the lunulae, Hythloday reveals how amazing it is that Utopians have experienced plague *only* twice in all of their history — a history longer than Britain's.[30] At the same time, attention is drawn to the fierceness of the visitation — it was so fierce, in fact, that it brought the population low enough to institute rules regarding the stabilization of the population. The plague made Utopians fear for the welfare of their nation. The plague had nearly usurped their control — a factor that any English man or woman would understand. The plague had also caused them to create contingency plans. In this, More's land of Utopia is shown to be flexible, still open to Bloch's Not Yet and unlikely to calcify into a dystopian state.

Although flawed, Utopians in the end inhabit "no place," the land that Davies envisioned where a king might safely hide his head. Utopian plague remains safely within parentheses. Even if Thomas More ultimately wrote *Utopia* as a bit of self-entertainment and not as a prescription for the nation, he did imagine a world grown out of his present conditions of plague-time and into a healthier future. By this one measure of better health and hope fulfilled, Thomas More offers us *eutopia* — a better alternative to plague-time England and perhaps a guide out of it.[31]

FOUR

Breath Infect Breath

✦

Plague in Shakespeare's *Timon of Athens*

In 1518 Thomas More utilized a set of plague orders to ensure that Oxford was free from plague before Henry VIII would arrive. In the same year, Henry VIII permitted the founding of the Royal College of Physicians. According to all scholars writing on the subject, both actions signal early interest in securing the nation's health. Yet neither action would result directly in improved conditions for the country as a whole. The orders Thomas More executed only served Henry VIII during that one outbreak. The founding of the Royal College was a move intended first to separate the learned from the unlearned physicians, determined by who was practicing Galenic medicine after the Italian models. No nationwide examination of healthcare had ever occurred, and a plan to preserve the health of England's citizens in plague-time was more than 50 years in the future.

After these first gestures at managing health, and before Elizabeth I's plague orders of 1578, plague visited England with virulent force in 1523, 1535, 1543, and 1563–1564. The last in this list was the first visitation in Elizabeth I's reign, and by all accounts it was one of the worst in the century. Adding to its virulence in Elizabeth's mind must have been her own near-death experience. Only a year before this visitation, in October of 1562, Elizabeth had caught and recovered from smallpox. She suffered a great deal during the illness. The event changed her life in many ways, as she began to wear the leaded makeup that would eventually cause her to lose her teeth and hair. She also considered her role as head of England. Her nation had no heir, yet she had come so close to death.

Like her father, she was aware of the great harm that might come to England were she killed without someone to take her place. It is only logical that her near-death experience with smallpox shaped her understanding of plague, when, within months after her recovery, it struck England with unusual force. Elizabeth had no coherent system for controlling its spread. None had been passed on to her, and there had not been a major visitation for two decades. But perhaps it was this visitation, which followed so closely upon her own affliction, that made it clear to Elizabeth that she and her people needed better protection. Perhaps this visitation demonstrated such a lack in Elizabeth's leadership that it forced her to think anew. The plague of 1563–1564 ushered in a new era of utopian thinking regarding improved health.

The visitation of 1563–1564 may also have given us the plays of William Shakespeare. Mary Shakespeare gave birth to William in April of 1564. Plague had visited London and was troubling other towns nearby. By July it had reached Stratford-upon-Avon, and we know it took lives only 300 yards from the home of Mary and John Shakespeare. The proximity of plague to the Shakespeares is noted by Park Honan, the only biographer working in the period who surpasses Barroll and Duncan-Jones in demonstrating the impact of plague on lives and literary works. Honan explains: "When her first son [William] was born, Mary Shakespeare's town lay in the path of the worst plague since the Black Death" (11). Mary had suffered from two previous miscarriages and assuring the survival of this son — in plague-time — was likely her highest priority and a source of influence on him:

> The emotional pressure of Mary's concern for William, her need for him to live, her prayers, tenderness, and watchfulness may be inferred from what we know of Stratford's suffering and Mary's previous experience of burying one or two of her girls. We have evidence of a situation, and of course must not suppose that we have access to her thoughts. But we need no psychological theory to explain a mother's ardent, sensible care for her son, day after day, when small children are dying. A pattern of Mary's special care for her son is also likely to have been set in these months. Her interest in him cannot have faded suddenly when Stratford was free of plague, and it is pertinent for us to think of his life ahead for a moment. William's confidence cannot be dissociated from the emotional support he must have found at home. (18)

Theater closings would also cause Shakespeare to question his livelihood, but perhaps the plague visitation of 1563–1564 established a home environment that was particularly nurturing for this budding poet and playwright.

By the time Shakespeare wrote *Timon of Athens*, he had become a prosperous man, able to establish himself quite handsomely in London and in Stratford. But this should not imply that he could easily ride out plague visitations. Instead, we find him in this period of his career rounding out a series of great tragedies, the compiling of which would exhaust any writer. He has also suffered the loss of his only son, the 11-year-old Hamnet, in 1596, and he knows there will be none to replace him. There will be no one to receive his legacy. And finally, the period from 1604 to 1611, during which he likely composed *Timon,* is one riddled with plague visitations and theater closings.[1] Work could not have come without suffering.

At the same time, we find Shakespeare writing at the end of a glorious national era. The humanist campaign initiated in England by Erasmus and Thomas More was over. The nation had seen the height of her glory come and go under Elizabeth. The new hope of England, James I, had shown himself less able to think about England's future prosperity and more apt to consider his own immediate problems. If we can view the humanist Renaissance and Elizabethan era in England as a rebirth for the nation, the first decade of the seventeenth century marked a postpartum depression. Individuals turned inward and toward the promise of personal gold mines acquired by foreign travel, money laundering, and alchemy. Plague would be no match, they hoped, for a golden man who could purchase his way to a better future. In this, many showed themselves entirely too susceptible to the fraudulent hope of which Ernst Bloch warns.[2]

Sir Walter Ralegh's 1595 voyage to Guiana in search of *El Dorado* was one of many ventures that enchanted English citizens with promises of wealth and health. His famous voyage ended in debt rather than in a surplus of gold, but his account of the venture made him nearly as famous as if he had brought back treasure. In one short passage from *The Discoverie of the Large, Rich, and Beautiful Empire of Guiana* (1596), Ralegh demonstrates why:

> Besides that we were not able to tarry and search the hills, for we had neither pioners, bars, sledges, nor wedges of Iron, to breake the ground, without which there is no working in mines: but we sawe all the hils with stones of the cullor of Gold and silver, and wee tried them to be no *Marquesite,* and therefore such as the Spanyardes call *El Madre de oro,* which is an undoubted assurance of the generall abundance; and my selfe saw the outside of many mines of the Sparre, which I know to be the same that all covet in this worlde.[3]

Although Ralegh did not secure this "Mother of Gold" for England's use, the promise of her bounty did establish English territories of the imagination.

Many others like George Chapman confirmed and embellished the account:

> Guiana, whose rich feet are mines of golde,
> Whose forehead knockes against the roofe of Starres,
> Stands on her tip-toes at faire *England* looking
> Kissing her hand, bowing her mightie breast
> And every signe of submission making. . . .
> . . . Whose barrennesse
> Is the true fruite of vertue, that may get,
> Beare and bring foorth anew in all perfection,
> What heretofore savage corruption held
> In barbarous *Chaos*; and in this affaire
> Become her father, mother, and her heire.[4]

Guiana calls willingly to Englishmen for rescue, occupation, exploration, and exploit. She longs for a civilized hand to bring out her true perfection. In return, the virgin Guiana becomes not only a child whom England can rule and but also a wealthy patron able to afford whatever England desires for herself. All it will take to tame Guiana, and thereby secure England, is the queen's support: "Then, most admired Soveraigne, let your breath / Go forth upon the waters, and create / A golden worlde in this our yron age" (30–32). The coupling of England and the virgin Guiana might begin with the queen's rectifying breath.

With such an *El Dorado*, one could purchase dominion over the known world, but just as important, one could cure all ailments. Medieval practitioners following Galenic prescriptions proclaimed that one could use gold in powdered, liquid, and solid form dropped in rainwater or wine to cure a variety of illnesses from eye-swellings to vomiting, heart conditions, and plague. Many scholars have written about gold's medicinal powers in the period. Because doctors at the time left plenty of testimony concerning gold's supremacy as a medicine, we can assess its growing popularity, which seemed to see its height at the end of the sixteenth and beginning of the seventeenth century.[5]

In 1602, Thomas Russel dedicated the *Diacatholicon Aureum or A generall powder of Gold, purging all offensive humours in mans bodie* to the "right worshipfull Doctors and professors of phisicke of the Colledge in London . . . (as well as to those at Oxford and Cambridge and) any cities or townes through this Realme of England."[6] In his treatise, Russel includes a poem entitled "G. P. Philosophiae chimisticae Studiosus," in which he explains,

> Each wit for wished health makes best invention:
> Some post a ship to fetch home Indian weed's.
> Some heape a masse of drugges, whose silly mixion
> May blindly hap to cure, yet oft the griefe it feeds.
> But all that love to trie some certaine remedie,
> Applie and taste this true, much labour'd misterie,
> Extracting health from Gold, in whose center,
> Of all foure element's, ther's perfect temper. (B)

Aware of the massive effort to improve the health of the nation, Russell recommends his gold-cure over the newfangled flights of fancy, for his remedy is time-tested and prescribed by "those two pillars of Phisicke . . . Hippocrates and Galen." By chapter 5, entitled "For what diseases this powder is good," Russel has listed "The Pestilence" as the last entry in a list of 55 diseases, which include "Loss of Memory," "Difficultie of Pissing," "Pissing of bloud," "for bringing down womens Flowers," and "Steerilitie or barrenness" (C–C2). Citing an enormous range of ailments, from things we would not call diseases to those most virulent even today, the list attests to the power gold possessed, at least over imaginations.

The same claims were being made years later, even though we know gold did not produce such cures. Francis Anthonie, a London doctor writing in 1616 felt compelled to write, in the Preface to *The Apologie, or Defence of a Verity heretofore published concerning a medicine called Aurum Potable,* that "The opinion of every excellent, both ancient, and moderne Physitions, concerning the virtue, power, efficacie, and use of Potable gold, is confessed in their owne writings: who do hold firme, that no Physition can well save the performing honour of his profession, without Potable gold, howsoever otherwise he be furnished with herbal Medicines."[7] Because gold was considered the mineral that contained within it all of the elements in perfect balance, people reasoned that it was the mineral most likely to bring the body's naturals into proportion, curing even the plague.

Those at the time who were beginning to challenge Galenic practices and consider Paracelsian chemical remedies only extended gold's power over minds. Where they differed is in prescribing the astrum or spirit of gold instead of its Galenic, powdered, liquid, or solid forms. Applying the astrum of gold to the body could cure the body's astrum. Gold was held to be the least putrefied of all metals, the one composed primarily of spirit and less so of matter. For this reason, it had more power than all other minerals to bring about health.

By the time of Ralegh's journey, the average person knew of such gold treatments. They were costly, and this only added to the allure of treasure tales that promised mother loads of gold in foreign lands or in alchemical labs.[8] Gold seemed an answer to plague-time and to a post-Renaissance malaise. When people are suffering, they are more apt to hope that the seemingly impossible can become reality, and they are willing to invest in that hope. The hope is then coinable if suitably packaged for audiences. Shakespeare, for example, made reference to Ralegh's venture in *Merry Wives of Windsor:* Jack Falstaff himself says of Mistress Page, "She is a / region in Guiana, all gold and bounty."[9] The average person could both appreciate and laugh at Falstaff's overstatement. According to Stephen W. May and A. L. Rowse, Shakespeare had also drawn on Ralegh's *Discoverie* in order to lend credibility to aspects of Othello's past and to the setting for *The Tempest. El Dorado* supplied Shakespeare with sources for tragedy, comedy, and romance.[10]

Ben Jonson had likewise written of quests for gold and new worlds. *Eastward Ho* (1605), written by Jonson, John Marston, and George Chapman (author of *"De Guiana"*), revolves around a fantasy trip to Virginia. The play increases the new world's appeal when Seagull the sailor describes it here:

> I tell thee, gold is more plentiful there than copper is with us; and for as much red copper as I can bring, I'll have thrice the weight in gold. Why, man, all their dripping-pans and their chamber-pots are pure gold; and all the chains with which they chain up their streets are massy gold; all the prisoners they take are fettered in gold.[11]

Seagull pushes the absurdities to their limits, matching Thomas More's Utopian chamber pots made of gold and adding golden irons for Virginia's prisoners.

On a slightly more serious note, Seagull shows Virginia as a place fit for a good man like Shakespeare's Gonzalo:

> Temperate and full of all sorts
> of excellent viands; wild boar is as common there as our
> tamest bacon is here; venison, as mutton. And then you
> shall live freely there, without sergeants, or courtiers, or
> lawyers, or intelligencers;
>
> . . . .
>
> Then for your means
> to advancement, there it is simple and not preposterously mixed.
> You may be an alderman there, and never be scavenger;
> You may be a nobleman, and never be a slave; you may
> come to preferment enough, and never be a pander; to riches
> and fortune enough, and have never the more villainy nor
> the less wit.
>
> (3.3. 34–51)

Even when placed within a comedy, the story of Guiana and her gold beckons.[12]

Of course, Shakespeare always reminded his audiences, as in *The Merchant of Venice* (1596–1597), "all that glisters is not gold" (2.7.65). The crucial action in *Comedy of Errors* (1592–1594) stems from the Antipholus brothers' trouble over the ownership of gold. From *Merchant of Venice* we learn that "gaudy gold" (3.2.101) can end one's marriage and one's life. In *Henry IV, Part II* (1598), Prince Hal accuses his father's crown,

> The care on thee depending
> Hath fed upon the body of my father;
> Therefore thou best of gold art worst of gold.
> Other, less fine in carat, is more precious,
> Preserving life in med'cine potable;
> But thou, most fine, most honour'd, most renown'd,
> Hath eat thy bearer up.
>
> (4.5.155–64)

In these plays, golden promises and heated desire for the substance nearly ruin its owners. Yet, gold does not quite thwart ultimate prosperity: the Antipholus brothers exit arm in arm; Portia saves the day, and Bassanio wins her (she is the golden treasure, wealthy and wise); and Hal inherits the golden crown. Real gold, if honestly earned, can make one prosperous.

In Shakespeare's most golden play, gold's poisonous nature overwhelms any medicinal quality it might possess. Written sometime between 1604 and 1611, when the plague had been continuously present in England, *Timon of Athens* is a retelling of Plutarch's *The Life of Timon of Athens*. To Plutarch's tale, Shakespeare added an extraordinary emphasis on the plague that follows from a lust for gold. In fact, the play contains the most uses of the word "gold" in Shakespeare's canon, with 36 mentions compared to *Comedy of Error*'s 19 and *Merchant of Venice*'s 15. At the same time, *Timon* has the second largest usage of "plague" behind only *Henry IV, Part I*.[13]

In *Timon*, the pairing of the terms "gold" and "plague" is more prevalent than in any other case, occurring with greater frequency than the pairing of "honor" and "shame" or "all" and "nothing" — sets of terms which have been considered indicative of the play's primary themes.[14] No one has examined plague and gold together, and I believe this oversight is largely due to a misreading of plague in the play. *Timon* is riddled with plague, but plague is most often interpreted as syphilis and used to support the claim that Timon suffers from sexual nausea.[15] By pairing gold and plague for examination, we gain new insight into a play that had seemed only to spawn commentary on capitalism or sexually transmitted disease. *Timon of Athens* is a greater tragedy if we take gold and plague in more literal terms, interpreted from within an era when golden promises persuaded men and women to pay dearly for their ill-placed hopes.

As the play opens we learn from the Athenians that their benefactor Timon is generous beyond reason:

> He pours it out. Plutus the god of gold
> Is but his steward. No meed but he repays
> Seven-fold above itself: no gift to him
> But breeds the giver a return exceeding
> All use of quittance.[16]

Timon possesses gold — lots of it. What is more, he enjoys giving it away. Like Seagull's Virginia that gives out gold for the copper paid, Timon's home becomes the most popular destination for men of Athens. He is their philosopher's stone.

The tragedy arises largely because Timon sees things differently and cannot imagine but that all are in agreement with him:

> We are born to do bene-
> fits; and what better or properer can we call our own
> than the riches of our friends? O what a precious
> comfort 'tis to have so many like brothers command-
> ing one another's fortunes.

> (1.2.102–06)

In his own eyes he is no philosopher's stone, no *El Dorado*. He is merely a good citizen, "born," as all are, "to do benefits" by making his wealth of communal advantage. If more men of Athens followed his model, a utopian community of shared wealth might emerge, as in More's *Utopia*. In fact, Timon wishes he were poorer so that he might more truly participate in such a community (1.2.97–99).

By the first act, then, the audience is already concerned for Timon, especially those of us who have read Shakespeare's later work, *The Tempest*. Fantasizing about his commonwealth, *The Tempest*'s Gonzalo is a nontragic Timon. There, in Gonzalo's utopia,

> All things in common nature should produce
> Without sweat or endeavor; treason, felony,
> Sword, pike knife, gun, or need of any engine
> Would I not have; but nature should bring forth
> Of its own kind, all foison, all abundance,
> To feed my innocent people.
> . . . .
> I would with such perfection govern, sir,
> T'excel the Golden Age.
>
> (2.1.160–69)

Gonzalo's dream reminds us of the Virginia of *Eastward Ho*. It is a land that is "t'excel" *El Dorado* and even Eden, perhaps, where people are all "innocent." In the mouth of an old man speaking to villains, however, such talk rings as harmless hopefulness or sweet naiveté, and Shakespeare leaves it at that.

Perhaps the hope of overleaping the fallen condition of humankind to a better society is permissible so long as it remains fuel for the dreams of old men. When it is not, it is more dangerous, more costly. In Timon's case such hope provides the material for jokes made by the ruling class: "It cannot hold, it will not," a Senator remarks, for "If I want gold, steal but a beggar's dog / And give it Timon — why, the dog coins gold" (2.1.4–6). Although the men around Timon know that his days as a veritable *El Dorado* are numbered, they dig him for more, and Timon continues to give without reserve. He wishes with each gift that he could give even more (1.2.219–20).

Here the hope most clearly and pitifully anticipates the tragedy. It is the vision of an *El Dorado* of the soul and of society that blinds a too-generous Timon to the truth: his friends are mere flatterers. As a human philosopher's stone, Timon is willing to "touch" all of his friends and turn them into himself — into *El Dorado*s. In return, they should come to his banquets, share conversation, and exchange love through gifts. The true sharing of wealth that Timon believed in and operated by would then appear. None in Athens would ever lack if all shared.

Inevitably, Timon needs money. He sends his servants to those friends, thinking they will act as he has, and even pleased that at last he can participate fully in the brotherhood he has created. Immediately and repeatedly, Timon is rejected. Slowly he is forced to realize, in the words of one of his trusted servants, that "they have all been touch'd and found base metal / For they have all denied him" (3.2.7–8). Rather than converting Athenians to golden friends, Timon's gold and belief in utopian sharing of resources have tainted them.

It takes nearly three acts of the play, but finally the Athenian greed touches and corrodes Timon's nature. As Paracelsus might have predicted, the tainted astrums of others imprint Timon's, rendering it in need of a corrective imprint from a pure astrum. In self-exile outside the city walls, he is a transmuted man, no longer hoping for a utopian brotherhood but for the death of all men. He renames himself *Misanthropos* (4.3.54), and shouts back to the city:

> Let me look back upon thee. O thou wall
> That girdles in those wolves, dive in the earth
> And fence not Athens! . . .
>
> . . . .
>
>   Piety and fear,

Religion to the gods, peace, justice, truth,
Domestic awe, night-rest and neighbourhood,
Instructions, manners, mysteries and trades,
Degrees, observances, customs and laws,
Decline to your confounding contraries;
And yet confusion live! Plagues incident to men,
Your potent and infectious fevers heap
On Athens ripe for stroke!

                                         (4.1.1–3, 16–23)

The utopia of Timon's former imaginings, Athens has earned
a dissolution into "confounding contraries" brought about by
"plagues incident to men" because it abused its one golden
citizen, the "noblest mind . . . that ever govern'd man"
(1.1.279–80).[17]

In fact, Athens is "ripe for stroke" by a series of plagues —
not just by one. The following scenes present that series of
blows stroke by stroke. Within moments of his self-exile from
Athens, Timon discovers the instrument by which he will
deliver Athens' death blow:

Destruction fang mankind! Earth, yield me roots.
[digging]
                        . . . .
                                         What is here?
Gold? Yellow, glittering, precious gold?
No, gods, I am no idle votarist.
Roots, you clear heavens! Thus much of this will make
Black, white; foul, fair; wrong, right;
Base, noble; old, young; coward, valiant.

                                         (4.3.23–30)

He has found that which brings about the "confounding contraries," that which transmutes one nature in to another and
the very object of his own downfall. A mountain of gold — it
will collapse the divisions of Genesis, of light and dark, night
and day, Heaven and Hell. It will act in the same manner as
plague, bringing "all out of tune."[18] Interestingly, it will reverse

the pattern established by Chapman in *De Guiana,* wherein one benefactor might bring perfection out of chaos by harnessing gold's healing power. It will also put to shame those who prescribed gold as a cure.

When Timon finds gold, he finds the medium through which to destroy a nation rather than usher in its golden age. First, he purchases the destruction of Athens by contributing to its most fierce enemy. Alcibiades is already leading a military campaign against Athens, and Timon decides to fund it: "Put up thy gold," Timon tells Alcibiades,

> Go on. Here's gold. Go on.
> Be as a planetary plague, when Jove
> Will o'er some high-vic'd city hang his poison
> In the sick air. Let not thy sword skip one.
> . . . .
> There's gold to pay thy soldiers.
> Make large confusion; and, thy fury spent,
> Confounded be thyself!
>
> (4.3.109–12, 128–30)

The gold is to pay for the first plague incident to humanity — war. Specifically, Alcibiades will become "a planetary plague" like Thomas Dekker's "Stalking Tamberlaine,"[19] the tyrant death who makes "large confusion," confounding the city. Old and young, men and women, rich and poor will perish together because they all contributed to Athens' "sick air." As in Sodom and Gomorrah, the rod of judgment will wipe out all who sin. In this case, the sin is against Timon's generosity, the persecutor is Timon, and Timon leaves no opening for the sinless to escape. As *Misanthropos,* Timon will use the plague as genocide and not as a rod of judgment intended to correct a people he considers his own.

But gold can purchase more than military might. With gold, Timon endows the second plague incident to man. When Alcibiades visits Timon, the prostitutes Timandra and Phrynia accompany him. Timon seeks to convert them into terrorists for his anti-Athenian campaign: "Plague all, / That your activity may defeat and quell / The source of all erection. There's more gold. / Do you damn others, and let this damn you, / And ditches grave you all!" (4.3.165–69).

By gold, Timon turns infected sex into a plague-like national scourge, a far greater act than giving syphilis to a few politicians. By giving gold to the prostitutes, Timon can deal Athens a second blow equal to that which Alcibiades will deliver. It is not a general sexual nausea that repulses Timon and pitches his madness to a higher level but rather nausea with respect to the human condition writ large.

Later he digs for roots to eat, and we see his misanthropy at its height. He begs Mother Earth to curse her children:

> Common mother, thou
> [digging]
>
> . . . .
>
> Yield him, who all the human sons do hate,
> From forth thy plenteous bosom, one poor root.
> Ensear thy fertile and conceptious womb;
> Let it no more bring out ingrateful man.
> Go great with tigers, dragons, wolves and bears;
> Teem with new monsters, whom thy upward face
> Hath to the marbled mansion all above
> Never presented.
>
> (4.3.180–95)

Timon again inverts the Paracelsian prayer, which would ask that Mother Earth's womb produce minerals and creatures each perfect in their microcosmic representation of a macrocosmic harmony. Instead, Timon wishes that the womb "teem with new monsters" — unnatural things that are naturally abhorrent to humankind. He envisions neither a utopia for humanity nor order in nature but rather a degeneration to chaos.

The plague that most disturbs Timon, we can see, are people themselves. What need for literal carbuncles and buboes when plague is other people? Timon is afflicted and cries out in pain when Apemantus the outcast visits. Before Timon's change, Apemantus had stood alone in railing against the injustice and inhumanity of Athens. Apemantus had been the city's crazed judge, but by this point in the play, Timon has outdone him. When Timon sees Apemantus approach, we expect he might embrace a like-minded companion, but instead he cries, "More man? Plague, plague!" (4.3.200). He refuses aid, and as Apemantus leaves, Timon curses him with more plague: "Yonder comes a poet and a painter. / The plague of company light upon thee!" (353–54). One visitation of human company follows another, mirroring the visitations at the beginning of the play — those Timon had loved. When the painter and poet arrive, we see that the plot has come full circle. The painter and the poet visit Timon only because they have heard that he found gold.

By this point in the play, it is clear that the individual and consecutive visitations of plague that Timon wishes upon Athens are delivered as a result of one single curse against humanity. To the degree that Timon embodies rage against humans, he also embodies plague. He greets part of his "plague of company," the poet and painter, and in an aside, he discloses his next plan:

> What a god's gold
> That he is worshipped in a baser temple
> Than where swine feed?
> Tis thou that rigg'st the bark and plough'st the foam,
> Settlest admired reverence in a slave;
> To thee be worship; and thy saints for aye
> Be crown'd with plagues, that thee alone obey.
> Fit I meet them.

> (5.1.46–53)

The poet and the painter are the men who have so worshipped a god of gold that they willingly follow him out into the wilderness beyond Athens. For this, Timon declares, they deserve to be canonized. Timon wishes to crown them with plagues, rather than with gold. He is most fit for that purpose: knowing well their martyrdom, he can justly reward them. He gives more gold and encourages them to spend it and spread the sin, thereby spreading the punishment.

Timon's fourth and final plague comes in literal form. Eventually the senators of Athens hear that Timon is plotting against them and that he has gold. This is a fine time to apologize, of course. They discover him, hoping to bring him back to Athens with them, and thereby take the first step toward appeasing a threatening Alcibiades. When he refuses, they ask if they might not at least deliver a message to the Athenians, and Timon proclaims that he "would send them back the plague, / Could I but catch it for them" (5.1.137–38). In this way Timon has not changed from the first act: he would gladly share what he possesses. He would happily catch the bubonic plague himself and die were he also able to infect Athenians with it. Certainly, and sadly, he is more likely to infect Athenians with plague than he was able to infect them with generosity.

Timon rests in the knowledge that he has other plagues on the way to Athens already, and he reminds the senators of this:

> Be Alcibiades your plague, you his,
> And last so long enough.
>
> . . . .
>
> What is amiss plague and infection mend!
> Graves only be men's works and death their gain;
> Sun, hide thy beams, Timon hath done his reign.
>
> (5.1.189–99, 221–23)

The plague will mend while it obliterates Athens, and if Timon has his wish, the sun will obey him and refuse to help purify the pestilent air.

Shortly thereafter, Timon dies and Alcibiades is poised to strike. He will carry out Timon's last wishes. The Senators scramble to save the city, and they ask Alcibiades for a compromise Timon never would have supported: "All have not offended. . . . By decimation and a tithed death / . . . take thou the destin'd tenth / . . . Let die the spotted" (5.4.33). The plague of war might only in this way touch those most clearly at fault.

Alcibiades must decide the fate of Athens, and he announces his verdict:

>   Dead
> Is noble Timon, of whose memory
> Hereafter more. Bring me into your city,
> And I will use the olive with my sword,
> Make war breed peace, make peace stint war, make each
> Prescribe to other, as each other's leech.
>
>   (5.4.79–84)

Alcibiades tempers his own role of plague so that in the end it brings peace. His punishment of Athens proves a more moderate leech-cure than genocide. What is more, Athens and Alcibiades will heal each other, so that all can live together in peace, better off than before the plague visitation.

This focus on the plague narratives in *Timon of Athens* makes explicit Timon's rage and the power of his curse on Athens, neither of which would have been as effective were it not for the gold funding them. The sources Shakespeare most likely consulted for the story of Timon — North's translation of Plutarch's "Life of Marcus Antonius" and "Life of Alcibiades" and Lucian's *Timon, or the Misanthrope* — affirm the originality of this depiction.[20] In his translation of Plutarch's "Life of Marcus Antonius," in which we find an account of Timon's life, North never links plague and gold. North used the word "plague" in translating Plutarch, but only in recording Timon's epitaph. Otherwise, there is no precedent in North for Timon's role as a golden man and then as a plague to Athens. In North, Timon functions more like the blind Tiresias whose power is in his words, not in his coins or in specific plague-curses.[21]

In the dialogue *Timon, or the Misanthrope*, Lucian only once emphasizes Timon's prophetic role coupling it with his plague curse. "Plague take you"[22] is Timon's reply to the visitation of Hermes, Riches, and Treasure, who come from Zeus to restore Timon's wealth. Such a curse or a word in an epitaph does not constitute a theme the way it does in Shakespeare's version, and when gold is mentioned in Lucian's dialogue, it is praised as in Jonson's *Volpone*. Lucian's Timon exclaims,

> O gold, thou fairest gift that comes to man. In very truth you stand out like blazing fire, not only by night but by day. Come to me, my precious pretty! Now I am convinced that Zeus once turned into gold, for what maid would not peon her boson and receive so beautiful a lover coming down through the roof in a shower? O Midas! O Croesus! O treasures of Delphi! How little worth you are beside Timon and the wealth of Timon! Yes, even the king of Persia is not a match for me.
>
> (2:385)

As a lover cataloguing his mistress, as Volpone, Lucian's Timon scorns the company of others in order to hoard his gold: gold is precious and to be held close, never paid out as plague-funds, never viewed as diseased.

The gold-funded plague and plague-bearing gold in Timon's story are unique to Shakespeare. His version of the life speaks to the dangers of believing that gold can single-handedly improve one's society in plague-time. It cannot heal humans who are flawed, and, in the end, one human cannot direct the course of plagues with will or cursing. One man's gold cannot bring about a community living in perfect brotherhood any better than it can bring about the utter obliteration of a society. But gold *can* make men think, vainly, that these impossibilities are possible. It can teach hard lessons about the danger of fraudulent hope. And, although plague can obliterate a city at the drop of a curse, it can also skip a town that seemed deserving of a blow. In these ways, Shakespeare has created a much more realistic affliction. In our first reading of the play, it seems that the plague functions primarily on a figurative level, as a threat of any other kind, from tempest to tornado. But when we put this play in its plague-time context, it becomes clear that plague is an intentional, distinct, and often literal force in the play.

The reason Timon selects a plague — a plague of many plagues all incident to men and not an earthquake, or war alone, or some other calamity — derives from Shakespeare's understanding of revenge, of the miasma theory for plague, and of his audience. The best revenge is to create a situation where the harms inflicted come back to harm the one doing the inflicting. Plague, with its infectious nature, is the only threat that behaves this way. It is the only threat large enough for Timon's revenge because it is within the air of Athens. When we first hear of Timon, it is through a discussion held by the Painter and Poet, who explain that flatterers like themselves surround Timon so that

> All those which were his fellows but of late,
> . . . .
> Follow his strides, his lobbies fill with tendance,
> Rain sacrificial whisperings in his ear
> make sacred even his stirrup, and through him
> Drink the free air.
>
> (1.1.80–84)

Timon's flatterers know that where Timon is concerned, the air about him is not only free but also coins gold. Those within breathing range of it grow wealthy, and healthy, although not wise.

When it comes time for them to help Timon, to resuscitate him so that he can pay his debt, they fail to do so. They shut out his servants who come to request aid, and at the news of the rejection, the exasperated Timon sputters "Give me breath, / I do beseech you, good my lords, keep on. . . . How goes the world, that I am thus encountered with clamorous demands of debt" (2.2.38–42). He learns slowly, as his loyal steward attempts to educate him,

> O my good lord, the world is but a word:
> Were it all yours to give it in a breath,
> How quickly were it gone.
>
> . . . .
>
> Great Timon, worthy, royal Timon?
> Ah, when the men are gone that buy this praise,
> The breath is gone whereof this praise is made.
> Feast-won, fast-lost. One cloud of winter show'rs,
> These flies are couch'd.
>
> (2.2.157–77)

These flies will by summer pester those near, a very sign of the plague. All this was caused by air first issued as a breath intended only to heal Athens.

The life-giving inspirations he shared with others are withheld, not redistributed, as they should be to breed social harmony. Kept within, they function as an inhalation trapped: they heat the system to a boil and without exhalation do not permit the body to cool. Eventually they will erupt. We see this happen with Timon, whose sick humors spew forth in a curse unique to this play within Shakespeare's canon: "Breath infect breath, / that their society, as their friendship, may / Be merely poison!" (4.1.30–32). Timon's choice of weapon is clear: that which delivers a suffering he knows from personal experience and that which always returns to taint its bearer.[23] He will infect all of humanity — himself included.

Clearly, *Timon of Athens* is a plague play, largely driven by the themes and language of pestilence, with its revenge plot, obvious scourge, attention to the air, and consideration of exile.[24] *Timon* also shares with more traditional utopian literature a depiction of two worlds in contrast: one, in which humans inhabit an infernal realm of plague and in which gold is misused; the other, where humans live peacefully, enjoying a surplus of gold because they know its true worth (most often using it as chamber pots and refusing to accept it from strangers). Then Shakespeare almost immediately inverts the topos, showing that dreams of a utopian community where all share wealth lead not to a utopia like More's but to the corruption of those generous men and Gonzalian lands. Shakespeare will not allow such hope to infect his audience. Timon's utopianism is exposed from the first act as false, unable to lead to an improved future.

This is not to say that Timon's original utopian dreaming causes the corruption. If it were the direct cause, we would not have a tragedy.[25] Timon's transmutation would be warranted, a long-overdue education. Instead we have the tragic tale of one who believed so much in his fellow men that he could not see who they really were. When Ernst Bloch explains that "even deception, if it is to be effective, must work with flatteringly and corruptly aroused hope" (1.5), he refers to deception intentionally created by one individual to practice upon another. Athenians took advantage of Timon's generosity, the tragic flaw that blinded him to the truth. Worse perhaps, Timon practiced upon himself. Corruptly arousing the hope of others is unfair if not evil, but arousing one's own hope without foundation is sad, when not tragic. Timon stands as a lesson originating in plague-time. By the time he wrote *Timon of Athens*, Shakespeare had learned this lesson. Gold and its promised powers had not prevented the death of his 11-year-old son Hamnet. Prosperity in the theater could not provide him with another son who would inherit the Shakespeare name and fortune. And gold certainly could not capture plague within utopian parentheses and render it harmless.

FIVE

What a Great Loss in Hope?

✦

Jonson's *The Alchemist*

Like Shakespeare, Benjamin Jonson had known loss of work during theater closings, and he was often away from his family during times of plague. Like Shakespeare, Ben Jonson suffered the loss of an only son. But unlike Shakespeare's losses, Jonson's were more literally at the hands of plague. It was bubonic plague that killed his son Ben in 1603. Within two years, his best friend John Roe also died of bubonic plague. He grieved for his son and for his friend in multiple forms, writing among them. In the years following each death, Jonson created some of the most poignant poems of grief in the English language. In the epigrams, we see in part what leads Rosalind Miles to concludes that Roe was "tailormade as a soulmate for Jonson" and why Herford and Simpson conclude in the notes to the Jonson's collected works that the poems written about Roe are "the most heartily affectionate of all of his epigrams."[1] The death touched off a fiery creative urge in Jonson.

It is possible that the deaths of his mother and stepfather further fueled that urge. If W. David Kay is correct in assuming that Jonson's mother is "the Rebecca Brett who was buried at St. Martins' on 9 September 1609, just 11 days after the death of Robert Brett,"[2] his stepfather, then it is possible that both of Jonson's parents, mother and stepfather, died in the plague. Their deaths, which were so close together, occurred during the time that theaters were closed, from 28 July 1608 to 7 December 1609. Among the many visitations occurring from 1604 to 1611, that of 1608–1609 left the very highest number of Londoners dead.[3] We do not have epigrams by Jonson on the death of his parents, and it is known that he was not particularly close to either; yet, whether or not they died of plague that year, we know plague did not spare Jonson's thoughts. After losing his son and John Roe, who by all accounts were the two people dearest in his life, Jonson would have developed a distinct impression of the scourge.

We see this impression in part through Jonson's play from 1610, *The Alchemist*. Above all others, this play is the most overtly pestilence-ridden. Only Tony Kushner's Tony Award winning *Angels in America* (1991) comes close to matching Jonson's play in the staging of infectious disease. Personally and professionally, plague had interfered with Jonson's life. It is no surprise that he stages a play in which utopian investments in plague-time leave their investors with nothing but hot air. We learn from the first lines of the play that no one here will tame the pestilence. It must ooze throughout the plot and touch the life of each character we see. It will also corrupt the audience, implicating us all. The play proper opens with a fart. The air of the viewing and performing space immediately ripens, and we desire to crack a window. But somehow, as the fume fuels the comedy, the dreaded stench amuses, revealing itself as a sign of the relationships on stage and their potential for producing abundant mirth.

As the prologue explains, the play is set in plague-time London. Master John Lovewit, owner of a home in London, has fled to the country and leaves Jeremy, his housekeeper, to watch over his home. With other plans in mind, Jeremy decides to turn plague-time and his master's fear of it to his advantage. He will con the citizens of London into believing he can deliver their dreams for a fee. Pairing up with Subtle, an alchemist, and Dol, his whore, Jeremy changes his name to Face, and the three set about to make a fortune. They will promise golden delights fit to make kings of commoners, fairy queens of prostitutes, and a healthful city out of plague-time London.

The inherent flaw in their program is the same exposed by Chaucer in *The Pardoner's Tale*: the promise of gold drives the team to compete. They have trouble getting along and when we first find them, they are disagreeing and threatening to turn each other in for the illegal adventure they agreed to make together. Subtle the alchemist replies to Jeremy's threats with that fart. Soon enough, Dol reminds the men that while they may be "laundering gold, and barbing it," they have together founded their own "republic."[4] They have joined together to turn their utopian dreams of a golden future into reality. By their arguing, they risk dissolving their new society in "civil war" (83), as Dol chastises them further:

> Shall it now be said
> You've made most courteous shift, to cozen yourselves?
> . . . .
> You will insult,
> And claim a primacy, in the divisions?
> You must be chief? As if you, only, had
> The power to project with? And the work
> Were not begun out of equality?
> The venture tripartite? All things in common?
> Without priority? S'death, you perpetual curs,
> Fall to your couples again
> . . . .
> Or by this hand, I shall grow factious too,
> And take my part, and quit you.
>
> (1.1.123–40)

Finally, Face and Subtle swear to "conform" (153) and follow Dol's advice to "labour, kindly, in the common work" (155). Of course, by this time, the audience knows that the trio's visions cannot fuel the labor necessary to build toward utopia. They will instead construct castles in the air — a foul, vaporous air at that.

Then the digging of gold begins, as one after another, men and women of London are duped. First Dapper, a young gallant, and then Drugger come to find their fortune. Simple tricks and games make these simple men easy prey, but the next visitor points out the dangerous blending of the genuine hope, naiveté, and desperation raging in plague-time. Sir Epicure Mammon enters, and in this one man we find the quest for the backyard *El Dorado*. The aptly named Subtle has conned Mammon into believing that gold is in his future, but that quite a lot of money will be required to initiate its growth. Subtle brags to Face:

> Methinks I see him entering ordinaries,
> Dispensing for the pox; and plaguey houses,
> Reaching his dose; walking Moorfields for lepers;
> And offering citizens' wives pomander-bracelets,
> As his preservative, made of the elixir;
> Searching the spittle, to make old bawds young;
> And the highways, for beggars, to make rich:
> I see no end of his labours. He will make
> Nature ashamed of her long sleep: when art,
> Who's but a step-dame, shall do more, than she,
> In her best love to mankind, ever could.
> If his dream last, he'll turn the age, to gold.
>
> (1.4.18–29)

Subtle imagines Mammon — "methinks I see him" — as saintly physician, potentially a messianic figure, ushering in a new world.[5] What is interesting is the beauty of this passage, which seems to charm even the cozener himself.

Mammon's incredible aspirations are indeed contagious, enrapturing even the audience. "Come on, sir," Mammon says to his companion Surly as they prepare to meet with Subtle:

> Now, set your foot on shore
> In *novo orbe;* here's the rich Peru:
> And there within, sir, are the golden mines,
> Great Solomon's Ophir! He was sailing to it,
> Three years, but we have reached it in ten months.
> This is the day, wherein, to all my friends,
> I will pronounce the happy word, be rich.
>
> (2.1.1–7)

Lines later, Mammon is still trying to convince the skeptical Surly,

> Do you think, I fable with you? I assure you,
> He that has once the flower of the sun,
> The perfect ruby, which we call elixir,
> . . . by its virtue,
> Can confer honour, love, respect, long life,
> Give safety, valour: yea, and victory,
> To whom he will. In eight, and twenty days,
> I'll make an old man, of fourscore, a child.
>
> (2.1.46–53)

Who would not hope Mammon is right? Who would not wish to be his friend if he did indeed possess the stone? With his riches come honor and love and eternal youth by means of a backyard *El Dorado* — ever at one's disposal.

Mammon's enthusiasm swells in seemingly credible and certainly enticing explanations of the stone's power:

> 'Tis the secret
> Of nature naturized 'gainst all infections,
> Cures all diseases, coming of all causes,
> A month's grief, in a day; a year's, in twelve;
> And, of what age soever, in a month

Past all the doses, of your drugging Doctors
I'll undertake, withal, to fright the plague
Out o' the kingdom, in three months.

(2.1.64–69)

While plague makes nature unnatural, the stone can "naturize nature" and remedy "all diseases." In Paracelsian style, so labeled by Mammon in later lines, the perfect astrum of the elixir will mend all astrums it encounters. His words become a positive contagion and enticing bait for a plague-time audience now primed to overlook the obvious.[6] Mammon continues his explanation: "I'll give away so much, unto my man, / shall serve th' whole city, with preservative, / Weekly, each house his dose, and at the rate —" (73–75). But Surly, his disbelieving companion, knows Mammon and chimes in, "As he that built the waterwork, does with water" (76). With this line, Surly reminds the audience that he who built the waterwork charged for the water upon which citizens became dependent. He believes Mammon is being taken.

Of course, we might not trust a character named Surly, but we know he is right, and after Mammon meets with Subtle, the false alchemist, he reveals his greed. Like Marlowe's Faustus, who exchanged his soul for delicacies from the orient, women, and gold — and who saw himself posting a plague dose — Mammon says to Face,

Now we ha' the med'cine.
My meat, shall all come in, in Indian shells,
Dishes of agate, set in gold, and studded,
With emeralds, sapphires, hyacinths, and rubies.
The tongues of carps, dormice, and camels' heels,
Boiled i' the spirit of Sol, and dissolved pearl,
(Apicius' diet, 'gainst the epilepsy)
And I will eat these broths, with spoons of amber,
Headed with diamond, and carbuncle.

(2.2.71–79)[7]

The "medicine" that might be used for curing plague and halting old age, Mammon will employ for strictly personal gain. His hypocrisy and greed are worse than Faustus's. At least Faustus wrestled with his conscience.

If this were Marlowe's play, it would be to the fires, and then some, with Mammon. But a satire to "better men" mends what is amiss in a manner that seems to let nature take its course. There is no room for a scene in which we hear Mammon screaming as devils drag him into Hell. Instead, Jonson allows Mammon and his contagious imagination to continue infecting others. And they do. Although we know that Mammon wishes to be like Solomon not only in gold but also in wives (50 a night with the elixir to increase his drive), his charm remains (2.2.34–39). We in the audience believe that Mammon may just coin gold. The question is for whom he will coin. If he cons enough people and turns all of their money over to Subtle in exchange for the philosopher's stone, then he will indeed be Subtle's golden man, the one ultimately to transmute all three poor residents of the Lovewit home into rich citizens.

Although the play's prologue has already informed us that the whole scheme will dissolve with the fume as the plague leaves town, an odd hope keeps us interested and convinces us along with the characters that positive transmutations will occur before our eyes — or at least that they are possible. It seems at points that Subtle is indeed the illustrious Doctor, a Paracelsian whose virtue is untainted, whose devotion to the art is pure. Mammon certainly believes this, describing Subtle's virtue to Surly: "He, honest wretch, / A notable, superstitious, good soul, / Has worn his knees bare, and his slippers bald, / With prayer, and fasting for it" (2.2.101–04). We vividly imagine with Mammon the devout old saint, and when we hear that saint speak, it seems confirmed.

Subtle chastises Mammon for his unrestrained, passionate eagerness displayed in Mammon's early visit to Subtle's door:

> Son, I doubt,
> You're covetous, that thus you meet your time
> I' the just point: prevent your day, at morning.
> This argues something, worthy of a fear
> Of importune, and carnal appetite.
> Take heed, you do not cause the blessing leave you,
> With your ungoverned haste. I should be sorry,
> To see my labours, now, e'en at perfection,
> Got by long watching, and large patience,
> Not prosper, where my love, and zeal hath placed 'em.
>
> (2.3.4–13)

Subtle plays the pure Paracelsian without flaw, and we somehow believe, if not in his transmutation from thief to alchemist, then in his ability to transform the minds of those who hear him. We of the audience also yearn to see this promised stone, and perhaps even to see Subtle's remarkable performance rewarded.

Dol also deserves gold — at least in the form of an Oscar for her roles as the Queen of Faerie under Subtle's conjuring control and as a lord's crazed sister sent to Subtle who promises to rid her of her prophetic frenzies. In each case, she entices her immediate audience of Dapper and Mammon, respectively. Like Subtle, she draws in the playgoers as well. We want to see her perform, and even though we never see her as Queen of Faerie, our imaginations fill in the blanks based on her ability to con Mammon. In some ways, we are as susceptible to her fraudulence as Mammon is.

Mammon is so taken with her in her role as crazed prophetess, that he promises to steal her away to a golden world of his own creation:

> We'll therefore go with all, my girl, and live
> In a free state; where we will eat our mullets,
> Soused in high-country wines, sup pheasants' eggs,
> And have our cockles, boiled in silver shells,
> Our shrimps to swim again, as when they lived,

In a rare butter, made of dolphins' milk,
Whose cream does look like opals; and, with these
Delicate meats, set ourselves high for pleasure,
And take us down again, and then renew
Our youth, and strength, with drinking the elixir,
And so enjoy a perpetuity
Of life, and lust.

(4.1.155–66)

Beautifully, deliciously, Mammon entices, and while certainly the audience knows to laugh, it cannot help but follow along, as if dreaming of sugarplums or the big rock candy mountain. This magical transmutation occurs with each character from Dapper and Drugger to Kastril, Dame Pliant his sister, and the Anabaptists Tribulation and Ananais. One by one, each is duped, but in the process each ascends to the very height of his or her hope, and we long to see the results.

We never do. All of the characters and their golden dreams turn into pumpkins with the departure of the plague from the city and the arrival of the homeowner Lovewit, who ends the venture tripartite and notes accurately that "The world's turned Bedlam" (5.3.53). What might have seemed like a world of possibilities is no more than madness, and when we step back from our experience of the play, this makes sense. After all, the action depended all along on the presence of the plague. Of course it was all madness. Of course we — the audience, the cozening trio, and the dupes — are better off now with the truth.

Or are we? Jonson immediately and effectively squelches even the immense hope of Mammon, to whom Lovewit, compassionately perhaps, asks, "What a great loss in hope have you sustained?" (5.5.75). Mammon reveals that the loss is far larger in scope: "Not I, the Commonwealth has" (76). In these words, Mammon shows himself more thoughtful and realistic than in all prior scenes, and Face, now returned to his identity as Jeremy, confirms Mammon's loss:

> Ay, he would ha' built
> The city new; and made a ditch about it
> Of silver, should have run with cream from Hogsden:
> That, every Sunday in Moorfields, the younkers,
> And tits, and tomboys should have fed on, *gratis*.[8]

There is no reason for Jeremy to lie now. Mammon does not even know that Jeremy is the same man, the man named Face who duped him, and Lovewit is not in a position to question or care one way or the other. What we hear is Mammon's sincere dream to improve the world, even if it was buried beneath the bolder desire to eat, drink, and fornicate beyond average ability. What we hear is hope exposed as false, hope lost. It is hard to recover from such loss, for it is the very same loss that results from the death of a loved one or from betrayal by a lifelong friend.

In the end, for every reason, it is clear that the vision of perfect physical and civic health will not and could never exist, and that the hope that fueled it was vaporous, infectious, and mean, a hope that steals from its host. Jonson succeeds in showing that all that glisters is not gold, and the price paid in its purchase can result not only in lost income but in the inability to imagine an improved future. Mathew Martin, among others, agrees that "Jonson dramatizes the failure of utopian imagination to be more than counterfeit gold," and that "the play's own anti-transformative poetics" highlight this exposure.[9] "Those who reply that Jonson's drama is worth the applause for its corrective, medicinal properties," Martin concludes, "assume the transformational logic that the play satirizes and accept Jonson's claim to be the true alchemist and his realist poetics the true philosopher's stone without considering that all alchemists make such claims" (407). Alan Dessen similarly sees at work a greedy, business-transaction mentality driving all characters in the play, including Lovewit: "The spoils, it is assumed, belong to the victor, not to the virtuous,"[10] leaving the audience "not . . . with a convenient ordering of the forces that have run wild for five acts but rather [it] plants the disturbing suggestion that, owing to our own culpability, there is only limited hope for improvement in the world outside the theatre" (137). Jonson squelches the hope in false promises and thereby effects the cure he had promised in the prologue:

> Our scene is London, 'cause we would make known,
> No country's mirth is better than our own,
> No clime breeds better matter, for your whore,
> Bawd, squire, imposter, many persons more,
> Whose manners, now called humours, feed the stage:
> And which have still been subject, for the rage
> Or spleen of comic writers. Though this pen
> Did never aim to grieve, but better men;
> Howe'er the age, he lives in, doth endure
> The vices that she breeds, above their cure.
> But, when the wholesome remedies are sweet,
> And, in their working, gain, and profit meet,
> He hopes to find no spirit so much diseased,
> But will, with such fair correctives be pleased.
>
> (5–18)

But when we read these lines carefully, we see something that critics have missed. The cure Jonson prescribes here is pleasing and the author, as doctor, operates with the aid of hope. Furthermore, Jonson determines that the setting for his play should be London not because there is so much vice within the city, but because "No country's mirth is better than our own." The venture and the outcome, then, depend on belief in "wholesome remedies" that are simultaneously "sweet." There is not for a minute here the suggestion that pain or confusion or any kind of self-flagellation will come upon audience members. They will instead find mirth, as Lovewit and his neighbors will.

Lovewit's mirth comes in the form of Dame Pliant, who had been nearly duped into a poor marriage by the pseudo-alchemists. Jeremy suggests to Lovewit that he marry Dame Pliant. A lonely widower, Lovewit is so happy with the prospect that he rewards Jeremy and forgets entirely about punishing him. With the reward money Lovewit gives him, Jeremy then tells his neighbors they will "feast . . . often, and invite new guests" (5.5.165). Mirth rules here in plague-time London. Lovewit's last lines confirm the same, as he thanks Jeremy:

> That master
> That had received such happiness by a servant,
> In such a widow, and with so much wealth,
> Were very ungrateful, if he would not be
> A little indulgent to that servant's wit,
> And help his fortune, though with some small strain
> Of his own candour. Therefore, gentlemen,
> And kind spectators, if I have outstripped
> An old man's gravity, or strict canon, think
> What a young wife, and a good brain may do:
> Stretch age's truth sometimes, and crack it too.
>
> (147–56)

Many have rightly seen Lovewit as implicated in the manipulations to the same extent that Jeremy and even the audience is. But one might also see Lovewit for his name's sake: a lover of wit, a man who would understand that crazy circumstances and vain dreams can sometimes bring about mirth — and mirth itself is medicinal, preserving a sound balance of the naturals.

Moreover, of all characters, Lovewit in the end gains the elixir that will stretch his life beyond its original measure. He does it neither by manipulation of others nor by exorbitant and naïve financial investment. We never see him lost in a realm of fancy, reciting how it is that he will secure the woman of his dreams. Instead, he profits by watching and by seizing an opportunity for prosperity as it manifests itself. In this way, he acts as the play's hero, one who balances self-profit with the betterment of others. He gains by marrying Dame Pliant, thus saving her from suffering. He rewards Jeremy for helping him find a young wife, and he presses no charges against anyone, happy that all has worked out. As the play closes, the period when the world seemed Bedlam is past. The plague is past. Life resumes, and Jonson leaves a bit of room for the possibility that on rare occasion, one can get lucky and be better for the visitation of plague.

If we examine Jonson's vision of his son's death, as recorded by William Drummond, and his last plague poem on the death of John Roe, we glimpse this thread of hope that critics who see Jonson only as a surly satirist have overlooked. In the vision of his son, Jonson sees the boy in bodily form, as if after the resurrection. And in the concluding poem on Roe's death, Jonson writes,

> ILe not offend thee with a vaine teare more,
>   Glad-mention'd *Roe*: thou art but gone before,
> Whither the world must follow. And I, now,
>   Breathe to expect my when, and make my how.
> Which if most gracious heaven grant like thine,
>   Who wets my grave, can be no friend of mine.[11]

In plague-time, one continues to breathe on, in expectation that leads through despair and even beyond death.

Like the characters in *The Alchemist* and the playgoers who watched in 1610, Jonson knew that plague could attack from within a nation and could strike within one's family. No place and no person could guarantee security from the literal disease or from its attendant sorrows. There would be no utopia for Jonson. And yet, in *The Alchemist*, Jonson delivers laughter along the way to a quintessentially comic ending. He delivers mirth, and by doing so, he provides his audience with a method of plague prevention recommended by Galenic physicians, housewives, and the writers of regimens alike.[12]

Six

Plague in the Foundation

✦

Building Toward *The New Atlantis*

During Francis Bacon's life, plague struck England multiple times with notable force: from 1569 to 1570; between 1574 and 1576, when Bacon was forced to retreat for seven months from the dangerous air of Cambridge where he was studying; from 1578 to 1579, when the Queen Elizabeth I issued the nation's first standard plague orders; in 1582, 1592–1593, 1603–1611, and from 1623 to 1625, just before the publication of *Sylva Sylvarum or The Natural History in Ten Centuries* and *New Atlantis* (1627).[1] Bacon understood the dangers of plague, having known of its presence in nearly every decade of his life.

We have evidence of his concern for his own health in letters from October of 1625, a plague year in which 20 percent of the population died in London: "Good Mr. Roger Palmer, I thank God, by means of the sweet air of the country, I have obtained some degree of health."[2] Bacon refers to an unrelated illness but is more clear about plague in his reply on the same day to the Queen of Bohemia:

> It may please your Majesty, I have received your Majesty's gracious letter from Mr. Secretary Morton, who is now a saint in heaven. It was at a time when the great desolation of the plague was in the city, and when myself was ill of a dangerous and tedious sickness. The first time that I found any degree of health, nothing came sooner to my mind, than to acknowledge your Majesty's great favour, by my most humble thanks. (*Works* 14:535–36)

Bacon escaped direct contact with plague, and after the visitation at Cambridge, it seems plague altered his activities only slightly. Lucky to avoid great loss during plague-time, Bacon had the money to escape from the city.

Nevertheless, plague could never have been far from his mind given the extent to which he writes of it in both his scientific and fictitious works, most of which precede the letters mentioned above. By examining the recurring appearance of bubonic plague in the writings of Francis Bacon, we can peer into a particular approach to natural philosophy, ascertain the degree to which Bacon promised to lead the nation into greater health, and consider his choice of genres when comparing him with others writing about plague and utopia.

Of particular note is Bacon's pairing of two texts — *Sylva Sylvarum: or The Natural History in Ten Centuries* and *The New Atlantis* — each dealing in part with plague. Bacon discusses bubonic plague in a total of seven chapters out of the ten making up *Sylva Sylvarum: or The Natural History in Ten Centuries* (from this point on, *The Natural History*). The significance of plague's prominence in this particular text is heightened by the important function served by *The Natural History* within Bacon's program of natural philosophy. Although current scholars generally view *The Advancement of Learning* as the quintessential Baconian treatise, Bacon would have disagreed. He viewed *The Natural History* as the base of his program, without which the larger structure of his natural philosophy could not stand. In the preface to that work, his editor Rawley explains:

> The scope which his lordship intendeth, is to write such a Natural History as may be fundamental to the erecting and building of a true philosophy. . . . For, having in this present work collected the materials for the building, and in his Novum Organum (of which his lordship is yet to publish a second part) set down the instruments and directions for the work; men shall now be wanting to themselves, if they raise not knowledge to that perfection whereof the nature of mortal men is capable. (2:336)

The Natural History catalogues truths of nature: observable, objective data tested over time and found to be universally sound. Most important is this claim of truth, as Rawley confirms: "I will conclude with an usual speech of his lordship's; That this work of his Natural History is the world as God made it, and not as men have made it; for that it hath nothing of imagination" (3:337). *The Natural History* contains nothing, according to Bacon and Rawley, but factual information, the building blocks of nature as God fashioned them for man. With these building blocks determined, Bacon believed, one could then assist God in a plan to rectify the world. The illustration from the 1658 edition of *The Natural History* depicts this partnership (see figure 7).

Bringing order to a massive collection of observations about the natural world, Bacon arranged them into the ten chapters. Called "centuries," each chapter focuses on a general category of natural history. Although we would not order natural history in this fashion now, we can see the early modern logic of the following progression, beginning with chapter 1, which covers the movement of all natural bodies and thus extends itself to observations of air, of digestion, and of disease. Chapters 2

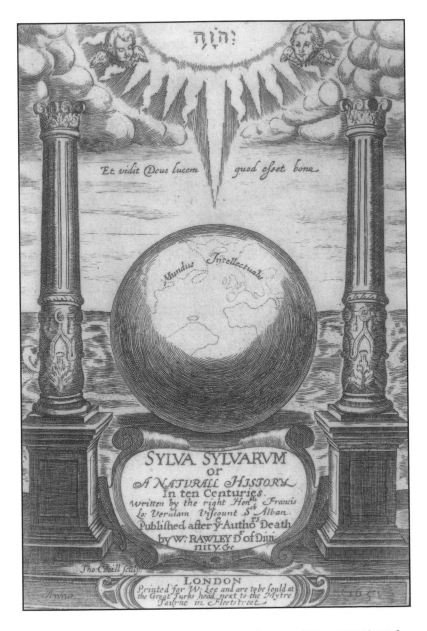

Figure 7. From Francis Bacon, *Sylva sylvarum* (Wing B328). Title
page. By permission of the Cambridge University Library.

and 3 report on vibration, particularly experienced as sound. Chapter 4 covers putrefaction and other metamorphoses of objects in nature, while 5 through 7 contain observations related to horticulture. In chapter 8, Bacon delineates the composition of natural, animate bodies found on earth, and in chapter 9, he records the effect of substances on inanimate bodies. In the last chapter, he records the power of the imagination, discussing the operation of sympathy and antipathy.

Each of the ten chapters then is divided into 100 separate observations, but what is most remarkable with respect to the present study is not the exhaustive endeavor (which we might also label exhausting) but rather the fact that the bubonic plague appears not only in a full seven of the ten chapters, but also in a number of observations within each. Within the very first chapter, in a section on disease, Bacon explains, "There is a secret way of cure (unpracticed) by assuetude of that which in itself hurteth. Poisons have been made, by some, familiar, as hath been said. Ordinary keepers of the sick of the plague are seldom infected" (2:366). Those who somehow grow accustomed to the disease might survive it. Bacon writes to record what he believes is a verifiable fact of nature. He does not write to judge or to prescribe what he calls "cures by custom." Only at one point does Bacon seem to prescribe a remedy: "there be airs," he writes in the last chapter, "which the physicians advise their patients to remove unto, in consumptions or upon recovery of long sicknesses. . . . It is noted also, that groves of bays do forbid pestilent airs; which was accounted a great cause of wholesome air of Antiochia" (2:937). Still, this is hardly a prescription but rather the recording of observations. There is a large difference between the two, but the essential point is that this is the only passage in all of Bacon's scientific texts that even hints at preventive measures for plague.

Bacon moves in chapter 3 to a discussion of nature's most virulent diseases: "There be some known diseases that are infectious; and others that are not. Those that are infectious are: First, such as are chiefly in the spirits, and not so much in the humors, and therefore pass easily from body to body; such are pestilences, lippitudes, and such like" (2:439). By assessing the various forms of infection, Bacon distinguishes plague from consumptions, leprosy, and the French pox (syphilis). This is crucial for his readers. We know after this point that when Bacon mentions plague or pestilence, he means a particular disease distinct from others and distinct in diagnosis from those that came before him. More specifically, we see that Bacon considers plague to affect the *spiritus*, a natural in the body much more directly influenced by air and easily communicated to others.

In chapter 4, Bacon paints a larger picture, how the "acceleration of putrefaction" (2:451) occurs: "The malignity of the infecting vapour daunteth the principal spirits, and maketh them fly and leave their regiment; and then the humours, flesh, and secondary spirits, do dissolve and break, as in an anarchy" (452). In this description, Bacon waxes dramatic, reminding us of More, Shakespeare, Jonson, and others who employed fiction, drama, and poetry as they sought the most suitable genre for capturing plague: "as in an anarchy," plague "brings all out of tune."[3] Few, until very recently, would accuse Bacon here of painting his political or literary agenda within the plague portrait. Plague is the focal point in its literal incarnation. The simile "as in an anarchy" serves to illustrate the literal affliction. That the plague might also be an apt metaphor for the state is not a primary concern here. While most scholars scramble to decipher the political implications of scientific treatises and plague texts, I believe such readings obscure the impressive efforts Bacon and others made to understand the literal disease.[4]

Continuing with his program for observing the literal manifestations of disease, Bacon moves quickly in the same chapter to establish the pattern for plague visitations as they differ from the occurrence of other diseases:

> It is commonly seen, that more are sick in the summer, and more die in the winter; except it be in pestilent diseases, which commonly reign in summer or autumn. The reason is, because diseases are bred (indeed) chiefly by heat; but then they are cured most by sweat and purge; which in the summer cometh on or is provoked more easily. As for pestilent diseases, the reason why most die of them in summer is because they are bred most in the summer; for otherwise those that are touched are in most danger in the winter. (2:468)

The causes and cures for many diseases are often supplied in the same season. Plague is an anomaly: true to its role as instigator of anarchy, it does not obey the rules.

It is even worse in England, where the land itself is more suited for plague:

> The general opinion is, that years hot and moist are most pestilent; upon the superficial ground that heat and moisture cause putrefaction. In England it is found not true; for many time there have been great plagues in dry years. Whereof the cause may be, for that drought, in the bodies of islanders habituate to moist airs, doth exasperate the humours, and maketh them more apt to putrefy or inflame: besides, it tainteth the waters (commonly), and maketh them less wholesome. (2:468)

While interpreting plague through a Galenic lens, Bacon is careful with his observations. He sees as Thomas More did that the region of the country is like the constitution of a particular body. Plague inhabits each differently, and we can hear Bacon speaking directly to an English audience reading the natural history of the world but also the natural history of their particular space within it. Plague acts differently than other diseases, and the English climate alone will not protect its citizens from violent visitation.

The remaining chapters of *The Natural History* appear to lend some reassurance through more observations by establishing — in Bacon's mind once and for all — the "certain signs" of plague. Chapter 7 provides these "prognostics of pestilential seasons":

> It was observed in the great plague of the last year, that there were seen, in divers ditches and low grounds about London, many toads that had tails two or three inches long at the least; whereas toads (usually) have no tails at all. Which argueth a great disposition to putrefaction in the soil and air. It is reported likewise, that roots (such as carrots and parsnips) are more sweet and luscious in infectious years than in other years. (554–55)

The style here remains rigorously scientific — "it was observed . . . which argueth . . . it is reported." The reassurance lies neither in the tone nor in the hypothesis, but in careful details a reader can trust and follow.

Chapter 8, the section entitled "Experiment Solitary Touching the Pestilential Years" continues to record signs with a reassuring specificity:

> It hath been noted that those years are pestilential and unwholesome, when there are great numbers of frogs, flies, locusts, &c. The cause is plain; for that those creatures being engendered of putrefaction, when they abound, shew a general disposition of the year, and constitution of the air, to diseases of putrefaction. And the same prognostic (as hath been said before) holdeth, if you find worms in oak-apples: for the constitution of the air appeareth more subtilly in any of these things, than to the sense of man. (576)

The more abstract concept of putrefaction from chapter 4 is made more clear here through detail.

Lest one think again that Bacon means only a general plague and not bubonic, he emphasizes the relationship between plague and all other diseases: "The lesser infections, of the small-pox, purple fevers, agues, in the summer precedent, and hovering all winter, do portend a great pestilence in the summer following; for putrefaction doth not rise to his height at once" (2:604). All signs of putrefaction — including all other diseases — might indicate a year ripe for plague.

Clearly the signs of plague were incredibly important, and all of chapter 9 is devoted to recording them in detail under the heading "Experiments in Consort Touching Perception in Bodies Insensible, Tending to Natural Divination or Subtile Trials." The more specific "prognostics of pestilential and unwholesome years" include "plenty of frogs, grasshoppers, flies, and the like creatures bred of putrefaction, [that] doth portend pestilential years" (602), as well as "great droughts in summer lasting till towards the end of August . . . [that] do portend a pestilent summer the year following" (603) — among many other indications. Readers today will be struck by the fact that Bacon has compiled an exhaustive list of plague-indicators he could not have observed entirely on his own. Not only are there too many of them, but they also appear to be copies of those made by others earlier.[5] It seems that those recording the certain signs of the pest borrowed from one another without determining the veracity for themselves and without specifying their sources.

We might wonder how Bacon could have called such a catalog of certain signes "observations" at all, let alone certain ones. Lisa Jardine explains in *Francis Bacon: Discovery and the Art of Discourse*:

> As the term is used today the scientist who believes a particular scientific theory (for instance that sound is transmitted by the air) contrives a test situation — an experiment — in which one outcome will be produced if the theory holds, and another if it is false. . . . Bacon's 'experiments' are not generally designed to test the truth or falsity of a scientific theory. Any observation illustrating some aspect of the topic under consideration which may prove useful in the future for *deriving* a theory is an experiment. Any observation of immediate practical benefit is an experiment.[6]

Such observations of "immediate practical benefit" might be found recorded in the Bible or in works by men such as Davies, Dekker, Bullein, and Paré. Repetition alone made a sign of plague made a more certain.

Bacon expands upon his "observations" to such an extent that he goes on to claim imagination, odor, and human intent as causes of the plague. Each of these could, after all, act upon the body, bringing about an imbalance in the spirits and humors. For example, Bacon tells us, "The most pernicious infection, next the plague, is the smell of the jail, when prisoners have been long and close and nastily kept" (2:646). Here, odors themselves are "infectious," and plague functions as the largest model for that kind of contagion, which is associated with social illness as well as physical. An odor, a sad letter causing one to mourn a loss, a fear grown to excess by the imagination — any one of these might weaken the body and make a person more susceptible to plague.

In chapter 10, plague metaphorically illustrates the infectious nature of imagination and men's susceptibility to others when sympathetic to them:

> As in infection and contagion from body to body (as the plague and the like) it is most certain that the infection is received (many times) by the body passive, but yet is by the strength and good disposition thereof repulsed and wrought out, before it be formed into a disease; so much more in impressions from mind to mind, or from spirit to spirit, the impression taketh, but is encountered and overcome by the mind and spirit, which is passive, before it work any manifest effect. And therefore they work most upon weak minds and spirits; as those of women, sick persons, superstitious and fearful persons, children and young creatures. (2:641)

Susceptibility to contagion can begin at any point — physical, intellectual, emotional, or spiritual. This helps to account for the vast number of certain signs and for Bacon's return, time and again, to plague as a constitutive building block in nature.

If we step back from the lists that seem to grow beyond proportion and beyond our current conception of what is scientific, then we find a pattern. What seems to be a conflation of too many coincidences in nature is based on a condition called *similitude*. Jardine explains with precision, quoting for support from *The Advancement of Learning*:

> What we might regard as a figurative resemblance is considered by Bacon to mark an essential resemblance. He insists that in many cases principles employing similar forms of words reveal an underlying general principle, rather than mere figurative resemblance: "Neither are all these things which I have mentioned, and others of this kind, only similitudes (as men of narrow observation may perhaps conceive them to be), but plainly the same footsteps of nature treading or printing upon different subjects and matters [IV.339]." (106)

In this way, plague in *The Natural History* functions both as a natural phenomenon in its own right and as a figure exemplifying the larger natural phenomenon of similitude. The literal and figurative manifestations of plague were for Bacon, as for More and all early modern thinkers, inextricably and physically bound, but it was Bacon who articulated the process and it was Bacon who wrote about plague as its best exemplification.

Given its prominence within *The Natural History*, it is not surprising to find the plague inhabiting its fictional companion, *The New Atlantis*. Rather than hearing about plague from observations largely independent of time and place, as in *The Natural History*, in *New Atlantis* we learn of a particular people and of their very specific measures for keeping plague at bay. The winds are the first antagonist in Bacon's tale: they blow the narrator and his crew off their course as they "sailed from Peru, (where we had continued by the space of one whole year), for China and Japan, by the South Sea" (3:129). The men, whom we later discover are English and Christians, find themselves unable to chart their position. They come upon a land inhabited by threatening people and decide to pass on before they eventually see another, which looks welcoming. This is the island of Bensalem, as they are later told, and although it appears welcoming, the inhabitants greet them with a serious warning: "Land ye not, none of you, and provide to be gone from this coast within sixteen days, except you have further time give you. Meanwhile, if you want fresh water, or victual, or help for your sick, or that your ship needeth repair, write down your wants, and you shall have that which belongeth to mercy" (3:130). The very first communication from the new world contains within it a preservative for the island.

The Bensalemites are right to protect themselves, even from our protagonists, because indeed the crew's "sick, they were many, and in very ill case; so that if they were not permitted to land, they ran in danger of their lives" (3:130). Three hours later, a "reverend man" in a turban came to inquire, "Are ye Christians?" (3:131). With the answer in the affirmative, and likely only because so, the people of the island begin to take steps to assist the narrator and his crew. In this concern first over health and then over religion, the Bensalemites remind us of the short, comic *A dialogue betuuixt a cittizen, and a poore countrey man and his wife,* written a decade later. The country wife, like the Bensalemites, similarly worries that the citizen from the city of London will infect her home, but when she discovers he is Christian, she decides to hold a feast for him.[7]

It is not quite so simple for Christians arriving on the island of Bensalem. They must take an oath, swearing that they are Christian, and then they will undergo quarantine, as a representative from the island explains: "My lord would have you know that it is not of pride, or greatness that he cometh not aboard your ship; but for that in your answer you declare that you have many sick amongst you, he was warned by the Conservator of Health of the city that he should keep a distance" (3:132). The lord of this new world obeys the Conservator of Health, who is in this sense the most important official on the island.

Respecting this warning, the crew, "bowed ourselves toward him and answered, 'We were his humble servants; and accounted for great honour and singular humanity towards us that which was already done; but hoped well that the nature of the sickness of our men was not infectious'" (3:132). They respect not only the warning but what is at stake: the lives of those on the island as well as their own. Soon, a notary holding a citrus fruit boards the ship, and the narrator explains, "he used it (as it seemed), for a preservative against infections," drawing disease from vessel and crew (3:132). This test and hopeful remedy for plague was one mentioned and likely employed often at the time, appearing for example in Jonson's *Volpone* (1605).[8]

The Bensalemite ruler demands further that the visitors, those "whole" and sick together, undergo three days in quarantine so that they do not infect the island with any disease. The quarantine, however, is highly civilized. The visitors are assured: "But let it not trouble you, nor do not think yourselves restrained, but rather left to your rest and ease. You shall want nothing; and there are six of our people appointed to attend you for any business you may have abroad" (3:133). They will reside in the spacious Strangers' House free of charge. The narrator is left to conclude, "God surely is manifest in this land," and any Londoner of the time would have agreed.

Quarantine was a much crueler and less effective program for crowd control in England, where entire households, including servants, were locked in the home together when any one individual in residence had plague. The practice was often criticized, as here, in Defoe's *Journal of the Plague Year*, when H.F., witness to London's calamity exclaims, "This is one of the Reasons why I believed then, and do believe still, that the shutting up Houses thus by Force, and restraining, or rather imprisoning People in their own Houses . . . was of little or no Service in the Whole; nay, I am of Opinion, it was rather hurtful, having forc'd those desperate People to wander abroad with the Plague upon them, who would otherwise have died quietly in their Beds" (61). Defoe concludes that the quarantine did as much, if not more, harm as it did good.

The strangers to Bensalem instead find luxury in their quarantine, lodging in "a fair and spacious house, built of brick, of somewhat a bluer colour than our brick; and with handsome windows, some of glass, some of a kind of cambric oiled" (3:133). Within the house were 19 chambers, "handsome and cheerful chambers, and furnished civilly" down the hall from an infirmary, so that as the crew members became well, they could easily be moved to lodge with those in health. This was a paradise by English standards, and by ours it looks to be a reasonable form of managed care that just about anyone might appreciate given its cost. It is free, paid for out of the Stranger's House fund that is rarely tapped. Moreover, it is built with the best materials available. "Especially brick," as Bacon informs us in *The Natural History*, is good for having "healthful air in their houses" (2:651). Within such dwellings, in such a country, the panic associated with quarantine does not exist. As Thomas More humanized hospitals, Bacon revolutionized the practices of quarantine by making them more hospitable.

In addition to civilized methods of crowd control, the Bensalemites also surpass the English in having established an organization of scientists from whom all advances in natural philosophy originate. Solomon's house would become a model for England's Royal Society decades later. After the narrator and his crew have cleared quarantine, they gain complete access to the island, and eventually the "father of Solomon's House" himself arranges for a meeting with the narrator. Looking the part of a wise wizard, the father, "was set upon a low throne richly adorned, and a rich cloth of state over his head, of blue satin embroidered. . . . He had on him a mantle with a cape, of the same fine black, fastened about him" (3:287). He is the man who best knows the ways of nature, the man whom Paracelsus might have called a magus. He peers into nature and understands her. By Paracelsian standards, he can see the correspondences in nature and prescribe accordingly. He explains, "the End of our Foundations is the knowledge of Causes, and secret motions of things; and the enlarging of the bounds of Human Empire, to the effecting of all things possible" (3:156). Control the motion of things and you can control plague's motion, which disturbs the motions of the spirits and causes anarchy.

Such diseases have little chance when so many motions are productively manipulated. For example, the magus tells his audience,

> we have a water, which we call water of Paradise, being by that we do it made very sovereign for health and prolongation of life. . . . We have also certain chambers, which we call chambers of health, where we qualify the air as we think good and proper for the cure of divers diseases, and preservation of health. We have also fair and large baths, of several mixtures, for the cure of diseases . . . and others for the confirming of it in strength of sinews, vital parts, and the very juice and substance of the body. (3:158)

Water that is pure and rooms fitted with clean air — the Bensalemites seem absolutely successful in controlling their external and internal environments.

To this end they keep the following:

> parks, and enclosures of all sorts, of beasts and birds; which we use not only for view or rareness, but likewise for dissections and trials, that thereby may be wrought upon the body of man. Wherein we find many strange effects; as continuing life in them, though divers parts, which you account vital, be perished and taken forth; resuscitating of some that seem dead in appearance, and the like. (3:159)

They claim they can keep animals alive even without vital organs and that they can bring them back from near dead. Perhaps humans are next on their list. If the vital parts of animals can be somehow found unnecessary for maintaining life, then one day Bensalemites may find that removal of infected parts of humans saves lives.

Until then, when such resuscitation in animals can be made to aid humans, the Bensalemites also have trees and flowers that

> come up and bear more speedily than by their natural course they do . . . many of them we so order, as they become of medicinal use . . . [along with] dispensatories or shops of medicines; wherein you may easily think, if we have such variety of plants, and living creatures, more than you have in Europe (for we know what you have), the simples, drugs, and ingredients of medicines, must likewise be in so much the greater variety. (3:159–60)

With respect to the available medicines, alone, Bensalemites have better methods for maintaining health than any other nation. Plague stands little chance with all fronts covered. The Bensalemites even manufacture odors, tastes, and heats, and they can proclaim, "You shall understand that there is not under the heavens so chaste a nation as this of Bensalem; nor so free from all pollution or foulness" (3:152).

Untested, untainted, as we would expect from a utopia, "it is the virgin of the world" (152), but this is only so because Bacon has followed Thomas More to a large extent. Bacon places plague in the similarly restrictive parentheses of constant prophylaxis. This is a virgin world ever on the verge of pollution from the outside, as indicated by the quarantine measures immediately applied when visitors come into port. Were there no threat of disease, and had the Bensalemites never experienced infectious disease, they would not have needed such comprehensive practices for health security. They would not declare these particular achievements highlights of their civilization.

As we learn in the closing section of the unfinished narrative, Bensalemites will continue to work very hard to safeguard their nation from those things they cannot eliminate:

> Lastly we have circuits or visits, of divers principal cities of the kingdom; where as it cometh to pass we do publish such new profitable inventions as we think good and we do also declare natural divinations of diseases, plagues, swarms of hurtful creatures, scarcity, tempest, earthquakes, great inundations, comets, temperature of the year, and divers other things; and we give counsel there-upon, what the people shall do for the prevention and remedy of them. (3:165)

Hardly at the point of being eliminated, plague is one of the many afflictions that the society must continuously assess. The result is a solid utopian system, made out of the same blocks of nature Bacon described with such care in *The Natural History*. More specifically, according to Arthur Johnston in the preface to a collection of Bacon's works,

> A list of the subjects investigated [in *New Atlantis*] shows the same interests as Bacon has in the *Sylva* — refrigeration, gardening and agriculture, longevity, brewing and baking, furnaces, light, music and sound, perfumes, engines and motion, deceits of the sense — and some others, such as microscopes and telescopes, clocks and perpetual motions, submarines and flying and mathematics.[9]

With the blocks of nature identified in *The Natural History*, Bacon builds New Atlantis. He does not entirely transform those blocks, but instead considers them in their best configuration. In the *New Atlantis*, then, we find crowd control and medicine in a blend of Galenic and Paracelsian theory, with men of science in Solomon's house concocting chemical compounds while also attending to the air. Both play a role in Bacon's program for the ultimate restoration of the world.

By putting *The Natural History* in motion, as it were, Bacon supplies an example of *similitude*. In *De Augmentis*, he explains:

> An object of sense always strikes the memory more forcibly and is more easily impressed upon it than an object of the intellect; insomuch that even brutes have their memory excited by sensible impressions; never by intellectual ones. And therefore you will more easily remember the image of a hunter pursuing a hare, of an apothecary arranging his boxes, of a pedant making a speech, of a boy repeating verses from memory, of a player acting on the stage, than the mere notions of invention, disposition, elocution, memory, and action.[10]

By reviewing this passage alone, we gain greater understanding both of similitude and of the effectiveness of pictorial contexts used to illustrate a more abstract principle. Utopia is just such an aid to memory, to learning, and to practice.

We also gain trust in the writer who can both postulate grand ideas and enact them before our eyes. James Stephens discusses Bacon's success in this regard: "Such pictures (from the Essays) reflect Bacon's feeling for similitude as a philosophical form. They contribute to the tone of a high and serious purpose and help to build an idea of the moral scientist in the reader's mind as one who 'reduces intellectual conceptions to sensible images.'"[11] Stephens is speaking of the essays, but we can apply this to Bacon's utopian work as well. Bacon helps to create and maintain an audience that trusts him. He sweetens his science with a styled context of "sensible images," which speak persuasively to readers.

The plague and all other natural phenomena are shown in the *New Atlantis* as integrated within the lives and works of the people. Scientific details are reassuringly few as opposed to those in *The Natural History*. They are equally slight on prevention and remedy and silent on cure, but again those were not Bacon's goals. By including the threat of plague, his work is tied securely to certain possibilities one might create out of the building blocks in *The Natural History*. Eventually, if the Bensalemites stay on course, they might reach an even greater level of perfection — one more closely approaching God's plan for the rejuvenation of nature.

We can confirm this intended, escalating path of improved health by reviewing the additional text that Bacon appended to the *New Atlantis* in its first publication, attached to *The Natural History*. The *Magnalia Naturae: Praecipue Quoad Usus Humanos* (Great Works of Nature for Use by Humans) is a list of what men can hope to achieve through science, and it is worth reviewing in its entirety. Here, however, I include only six of the 33 great works, and I have numbered them to indicate their order:

1) The prolongation of life.
2) The restitution of youth in some degree.
3) The retardation of age.
4) The curing of diseases counted incurable.
14) Making of new species.
30) Natural divinations.

(3:167–68) [12]

Bacon does not include the elimination of diseases counted incurable but rather their cure. He does not claim that his program will lead to eternal life of the physical body, but it will provide for a return to youth "in some degree." To make bolder claims would render his science pure fiction. His utopian strategy is to manage what is within the realm of the possible.

The Bensalemites are almost there, but they have not made it yet. Of the 33 goals Bacon lists, his utopians mention mastery of 17, just over half. The numbers that follow in parentheses coincide with those in the *Magnalia Naturae*, while the numbers in brackets indicate the pages of the *New Atlantis* where the particular outcome is mentioned. They have prolonged life (1 [3:158]); altered existing species and made new ones (13, 14 [159]); accelerated maturations, clarifications, putrefaction, and germination (19, 21–23 [157–59]); and conducted natural divinations (30 [166]), among other things. They have not, obviously, brought about "the curing of diseases counted incurable" (3), although they do claim to "cure divers diseases" [158]. They do not claim to bring about a "restitution of youth" in humans (2), a "mitigation of pain" (5), or the "altering of complexions," statures, or features in humans (9–11); nor have they mastered the ability for humans to alter bodies by force of imagination alone (18).

The importance of this list is immeasurable, and surprisingly, no study of it exists. I believe it answers once and for all the question regarding Bensalem: to what extent does Bensalem provide a complete picture of Bacon's goal for humanity? The answer is "half way", and this poses a challenge for those wanting to prove that Bensalem is a perfect model of the Edenic life humans can attain through Baconian science. Bensalemites might one day eliminate threats to health, but for now they must monitor nature with steadfast devotion and serious inquiry. They are aware of the stakes, as they watch their borders. Bensalemites do not yet recreate themselves in peace to the extent that More's Utopians do. But then, More's Utopians were indeed of a prior era in utopian and plague literature. They maintained a nearly closed system within which they regulated plague and their utopian projects internally.

By Bacon's time, it took more effort to capture plague in parentheses, and we could easily say that although Bacon believed it might be done, he recognized the effort would be enormous. He faced a plague that threatened from outside as well as from inside, and in this way, his conception of plague is more realistic than Thomas More's. Bacon did not understand contagion as we do, but he understood that no matter how balanced one's naturals or one's nation was, a threat from the outside could throw all out of tune. Prevention would require a regimen for individual bodies but also constant monitoring of nature and of one's physical and national borders.

This necessitates a Commissioner of Health, an occupation unnecessary in More's *Utopia*, but one that has quite a future with current incarnations grown to international proportions. If the World Health Organization (WHO) decides to issue a travel advisory for a particular city, as it did for Toronto in the summer of 2003, governments carry out the WHO's recommendations, and individuals obey.

At the same time, while Bacon's utopians must work harder to control disease, their hope in a cure exists, as it cannot for More's utopians. In fact, only the belief in a plague-cure held by *The Alchemist's* Epicure Mammon displays greater hope, and it is fraudulent. Bacon's hope — though unrealized in his lifetime — is the mother of our own: a belief that through careful observation of nature, we can understand and control her for our greater good. Although many of us question whether or not such hope in the increased control over nature is healthy from an ecological standpoint, it was, nevertheless, an important step toward the ultimate identification of bacteria and, as Bacon hoped, a cure for plague.

SEVEN

Fly from that Pestilent Destruction

Margaret Cavendish's Prescriptions

A Royalist, Margaret Cavendish was the Duchess of New-castle, formerly a maid in Henrietta Maria's court, who met her husband William in France during their mutual Civil War exiles. The pair created plays, poetry, drama, scientific trea-tises, biographies, and active social and intellectual lives rather than children. By the end of her career, having earned a reason-able reputation among members of the scientific community and notoriety among the inhabitants of London, Cavendish had cultivated a public persona of the crazed artist and was therefore known by some as Mad Madge. She was not unusual, however, in fearing the plague and in viewing the power of nature in light of its threats. Like Francis Bacon, Cavendish worked diligently to represent the literal affliction of bubonic plague in her many treatises on natural philosophy. Like Bacon, she also paired with one such treatise a fictional account of another world that was in many ways superior to England, but which also struggled to understand bubonic plague.

Even more interesting is that while Francis Bacon's treatment of plague is largely contained within *The Natural History* and *New Atlantis*, Margaret Cavendish includes bubonic plague in the majority of her nondramatic works. While Bacon's writings reveal an assessment of plague fashioned within one period of his lifetime, Cavendish's many treatments vary over decades. We can track her changing views through her literary corpus. When we do, we find that hand in hand with her growing knowledge of natural philosophy is an increasing understanding of and concern over the bubonic plague. The shift suggests a key to her development as a natural philosopher and as a writer, permitting us to capture in miniature her maturing understanding of the human condition.

At 30 years of age, after nearly a decade in exile during the Civil War and Interregnum, Margaret Cavendish returned to London with her husband's brother in order to regain possession of some of the family estates taken during the war. By the end of her two-year stay, she left, having failed in her original objective for the venture but having discovered her vocation. Before she left England for Antwerp to rejoin William, she had published a book of poetry, *Poems and Fancies* (1653), and written herself into history. As Katie Whitaker reports in *Mad Madge: The Extraordinary Life of Margaret Cavendish, Duchess of Newcastle, the First Woman to Live by her Pen*, "this was the first book of English poetry to be deliberately published by a woman under her own name," and it was her first commentary on plague.[1]

In "A World in an Eare-Ring," the plague inhabits the tiniest of places:

> AN *Eare-ring round* may well a *Zodiacke* bee,
> Where in a *Sun* goeth round, and we not see.
>
> . . . .

There *Night,* and *Day,* and *Heat,* and *Cold,* and so
May *Life,* and *Death,* and *Young,* and *Old,* still grow,
Thus *Youth* may spring, and severall *Ages* dye,
Great *Plagues* may be, and no *Infections* nigh.

· · · · · · · ·

There *Governours* do rule, and *Kings* do Reigne,
And *Battels* fought, where many may be slaine

· · · · · · · ·

There may be *dancing* all Night at a *Ball,*
And yet the *Eare* be not disturb'd at all.[2]

This tiny world in an earring is one of the many millions of microcosms, all of which, Cavendish suggests, come complete with kings, dancing, war, and plague. A global rather than a universal scourge, the plague is contained within the world of that earring, and it cannot disturb the lady's ear. Within the parenthetical of the earring, as it were, plague threatens limited numbers and elicits no fear from Cavendish's readers.

Within the same year, Cavendish finished her second work, the *Philosophical Fancies.*[3] In this extension of her *Poems,* Cavendish focused on her theories of natural philosophy from "The Unity of Nature" and "Of Thin, and Thick Matter" to "Of the Senses" and "Of the Sun." Concluding that in this short treatise there had not been enough time for her to discuss other subjects of equal interest, she notes those she would like to have covered:

What Motion makes the Aire pestilent, and how it comes to change into severall diseases? And whether Diseases are just alike, and whether they differ as the Faces of Men do? Why some Figures are apt to some Diseases, and others not? And why some kind of Drugs, or Cordialls, will worke on some Diseases, and not on others? And why some Drugs have strong effects upon some Humours, and not upon others? And why Physicke should purge, and how some Cordials will rectifie the disorderly Motion in a distemper'd Figure? (G5)

Already imagining her next work, Cavendish suggests that although she wonders at these things, here she "will give [her] Readers so much Light, as to guesse what [her] Fancies would have beene at" (G7).

Begun immediately thereafter, upon her return from London to Antwerp, *The World's Olio* is the first of her many efforts to answer those questions.[4] Although it would take her two years to publish the work, we can see its affinity with the ideas initiated in *Poems and Fancies*, particularly with respect to plague. In the *Olio*, her decidedly miscellaneous reflections on the human condition, she explains in more scientific and perhaps realistic terms the subject of plague's proportions: "The Diseases in the Summer" include

> Plagues, by reason the Heat inflames those Malignant and Corrupted Humours that the Winter hath bred by Obstructions, like Houses that are musty, and fusty, and smoky, and foul, for want of Air to sweeten them; and full of Spiders, and Cobwebs, and Flyes, and Moths, bred from the dusty dirty Filth therein, for want of Vent to purge them, for the Winter shuts up all the Windows and Dores, which are the Pores; likewise the Blood corrupts, and the Body is apt to rot, like Linnen, that is laid up damp, or in a moyst place. (162)

Here plague visitations occur, as cobwebs do before spring cleaning. The description reminds us of William Bullein's account of plague's certain signs. Suited to a Galenic diagnosis of imbalanced humors, plague in Cavendish's *Olio* is a rather mild imbalance within the system, not much worse than a musty home in need of seasonal purging.

From her first three works, we can perceive a concern regarding the plague's place in human lives, but it is minimal. Whether Cavendish depicts plague as within the earring or as a mustiness awaiting ventilation, these plagues do not evoke fear in the narrator or the reader. They will pass almost unnoticed, with little or no action required on the part of the witness. With respect to Cavendish's selection of genre, however, we see a different and powerful trend emerge. By her analogy showing that "Malignant and corrupted Humors that the Winter hath bred by Obstructions" are like "Houses that are musty, and fusty, and smoky, and foul," Cavendish unites scientific observation and literary creation.

Cavendish would continue in nearly all of her nondramatic writings to blend science and fiction to a greater extent than others before her. In 1655, the same year in which she published *The World's Olio*, Cavendish published her first major work entirely devoted to the subject of natural philosophy. Originally intended as a correction and expansion of her ideas from *The Philosophical Fancies*, her new work, entitled *Philosophical and Physical Opinions*, warranted its new title. Most prominent in the added material, Cavendish's treatment of disease grew to include multiple chapters. In "Of the expelling malignity to the outward parts of the body," Cavendish suggests that "the reason why malignant diseases, as the plague, or purples, or small pox, measles, or the like; there break forth spots, swelling scabs, or whelks, is by the power of expelling motion."[5] She then attributes this motion to "too much humor, obstructing the body therewith, so there is too much motion to work regularly therein, and being against the natural constitution to have so much humour, and motion, it produceth violent sickness, working to the destruction, and not to the maintenance of the body." Here, Cavendish takes on a different voice than we hear in her previous work. It is a more distant, objective, and what we might call scientific voice.

Although she does not question whether diseases are all the same or have different faces, as she did earlier, Cavendish sets the stage for doing so when she discusses in "The knowledge of diseases,"

> It is not sufficient for Physitians to study the names of diseases, and to know onely so much as to distinguish one kinde of disease from another, as we should distinguish man from

> beast, or so, as a horse from a cow, or as that horse is a barbe, or
> a coarser, or a genet, or a Turk, or an Arabian, but that this
> barbe, is not that barbe, or this genet is not that genet, and the
> like. (169)

This cute example is quite astute, as Cavendish makes clear
that within the symptom of fevers there are sets and within
those there are individuals, and a doctor must be familiar with
each one.

By the time Cavendish would revise her *Philosophical and
Physical Opinion* (hereafter *Philosophical and Physical*) again
in 1663, much had changed in her life, and her writing was
coming to match her maturity. After the Restoration, she and
her husband had returned to England where she wrote and
published a collection of plays. Her mind could never have
been far from her desire to understand the natural world in
general and disease in particular. In a chapter on "Spotted
Feavers, Especially the Spotted Plague," Cavendish begins to
answer the question she posed in *The Philosophical Fancies*
more than a decade earlier, "whether Diseases are just alike,
and whether they differ as the Faces of men do?":

> Those Diseases that are named the Purples, or Spotted Feaver,
> and Plague, are not only caused by a Superfluity of Humours,
> or a Corruption of Humours, but an Inflammation of the Vital
> parts, and Vital spirits, as also of Loose humours, as Blood and
> Choler, which for the most part causeth a Total ruine of the
> Whole body, and where one Patient Lives, Hundreds Dye in
> those Violent Diseases.[6]

Cavendish displays a clearly Galenic understanding of plague
like that in *The World's Olio*. But she does suggest that not
all diseases are alike.

Then, she describes the sign of certain death by plague, a
disease with an unusual face: "As for the Disease of the Plague,
when that Disease breaks out into Round, Dark, or Bloody
Spots, it is a sign of Certain Death, for I never Heard that any

Lived after those Spots were in the Flesh, those Spots showing a Total Infection throughout the Body, and Parts of the Body" (*Philosophical and Physical*, 338). In her willingness to describe vividly the signs of the illness, Cavendish shows that her knowledge of the disease is more than book-bound. She envisions and captures the sores in writing. In doing so, she takes a step beyond the others in this study. She causes her readers to witness the suffering body.

Then she takes another step in her empathetic witnessing: "Were I so diseased, if I had any time of Life, as three or four Hours, I would Bleed in many Several Veins at One time, especially those Veins under my Tongue; for those Veins do most generally Draw from all parts of the Body; also I would be Let Blood in my Arms and Legs immediately after those mouth-veins, for if any thing will Cure a Spotted Plague, it must be by Sudden and Extraordinary Evacuations, because the Disease is Violent, and causes a Sudden Destruction" (*Philosophical and Physical*, 339). A violent purging might cure a violent plague, she suggests. And if she had only a few hours to live, having already found the spots upon her, then why not try? Here Cavendish supplies us with an interesting combination of scientific observation, the kind of which Bacon might approve, followed by her own projections: "were I so diseased." She records but then guesses, observes objectively but then enters herself as a hypothetical example. Imaginatively envisioning herself the plague victim, she extends an invitation to the reader to consider her diseased body, as if she were the subject of anatomy in a textbook such as Thomson's *Loimotia, or, The pest anatomized* published in 1666 (see figure 8). In her willingness to bridge the gap between victim and witness, Cavendish stands alone among the others in this study.[7]

The notable change in the rigor of Cavendish's treatment of plague and of other subjects pales in comparison to that which was to follow. By 1666, Cavendish had published two collections of letters — one primarily social and another more

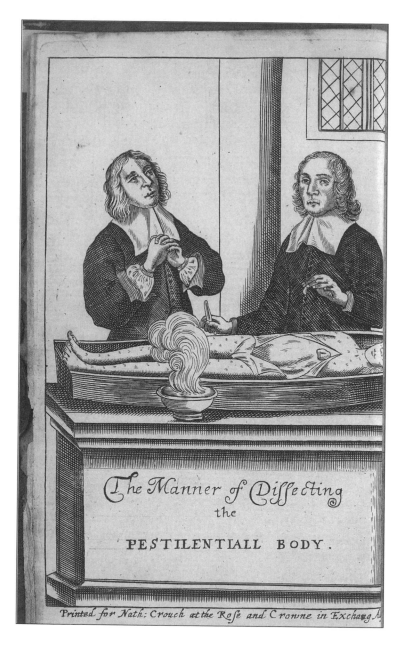

The Manner of Dissecting the

PESTILENTIALL BODY.

Printed for Nath: Crouch at the Rose and Crowne in Exchang A

Figure 8. From George Thomson, *Loimotomia* (Wing T1027).
Facing title page. By permission of the Huntington Library.

scientific.[8] By 1666, Cavendish had also been around the block socially and within the scientific community to the extent that she had developed her own understanding of nature — an understanding fully informed by, and yet standing distinct from, the finest minds of the day, from Hobbes to Boyle and Descartes whom she had entertained in London and abroad.[9] She no longer feared that her writing lacked power or that she would somehow bring trouble to her family through writing. By 1666, Cavendish had also lived through the last major plague in England. The change in just three years is dramatic, as evidenced in her treatment of plague in what has become her most famous and unusual publication, *The Description of a New World Called the Blazing World* (hereafter *The Blazing World*).

As a utopia, *The Blazing World* has a plot, making it easier to follow than the majority of her nondramatic works. It is also relatively short, and for these reasons it finds its way into anthologies and onto course syllabi. However, this work that appears to many as the highlight of her literary corpus was not at first intended for publication by itself. In fact, the 1666 volume in which it was contained emphasizes the *other* work, as indicated by the title: *Observations Upon Experimental Philosophy: To Which is added, the Description of a New Blazing World* (hereafter *The Observations*).

Comparison of the plague passages in each text shows exactly how one might read the two larger narratives as companion works, and how such a reading can and should be extended to other subjects. In the case of the plague passages, not a single line of the lengthy plague narrative in *The Observations* is repeated in *The Blazing World*. One can splice together the two narratives, and the information on plague grows without being duplicated. It is also interesting to keep in mind the difference between treatment of the plague here and that in her previous works. Here plague emerges as a distinct threat standing alone. In *The Blazing World* no other disease is discussed at length, and in the revision of *The Observations,* Cavendish devotes a chapter to plague. She gives no other disease such attention, but it is even more revealing that she places "25. Of the Plague" in a special section of *The Observations* entitled "Further Observations upon Experimental Philosophy, reflecting withal upon some Principal Subjects in Contemplative Philosophy." She inserts it between chapters "24. Of Fermentation" and "26. Of Respiration." In this position, the subject of plague is elevated not only above the consideration of all other diseases, but also above her own estimation of the scourge only three years earlier. The plague is now a constitutive force of nature side by side with fermentation and respiration, the very processes that begin death and deliver life.

The first discussion of plague in *The Blazing World* concludes a lengthy exchange between the Empress, originally a newcomer to the land, and the teams of natural philosophers she has appointed to ensure the prosperity of the realm:

> Lastly, her Majesty had some conferences with the Galenic physicians about several diseases, and amongst the rest, desired to know the cause and nature of . . . the spotted plague. They answered, that . . . the spotted plague was a gangrene of the vital parts, and as the gangrene of outward parts did strike inwardly; so the gangrene of inward parts, did break forth outwardly; which is the cause, said they, that as soon as the spots appear, death follows; for then it is an infallible sign, that the body is throughout infected with a gangrene, which is a spreading evil; but some gangrenes do spread more suddenly than others, and of all sorts of gangrenes, the plaguey-gangrene is the most infectious; for other gangrenes infect but the next adjoining parts of one particular body, and having killed that same creature, go no further, but cease; whenas, the gangrene of the plague, infects not only the adjoining parts of one particular creature, but also those that are distant; that is, one particular body infects another, and so breeds a universal contagion.[10]

Although the Empress also has at her command a group of chemists, of experimental philosophers, and natural philosophers, she selects her Galenic physicians to discourse upon plague. Of particular note is the degree to which the Empress appears to favor the Galenic practitioners, particularly over the chemists, whom she disbands, refusing to allow them to practice further.[11]

In a presentation free from embellishment — one that Bacon might have appreciated — the Galenic practitioners inform us that the plague is an internal gangrene of the vital parts that spreads outwards. But then they provide a literary and utopian perspective: plague in the land of the *Blazing World* is a "spreading evil" that "breeds a universal contagion." A universal contagion can travel from one world to another. What Cavendish makes clear is that plague is no longer a disease of the summer, the simple reaction of humors to a lack of purging, as she stated in 1653; nor is it isolated within one world, as in the earring. Cavendish sees the plague in its universal dimensions, an incurable "spreading evil."

Such a disease, clearly differing from others and presenting the most sinister face of all, warrants additional attention in *The Blazing World* and in *Observations,* where Cavendish explains,

> Concerning the Spotted-Plague, it proceeds from a general irregularity of Dissolving-motions, which cause a general Gangrene of all the Body; and to find a Cure for this Disease, is as difficult, as to find the Philosophers-Stone; for, though many pretend to cure it, yet none has as yet performed it; what may be done hereafter, I know not; but I doubt they will be more able to raise a man from the dead, or renew old age, and change it into Youth, than do it. (90)

The land of the Blazing World is a place where restorative beds can keep inhabitants living to their 401st birthday. It makes sense to wonder why the advanced practitioners of such a world cannot think through a remedy for plague. But Cavendish supplies the answer here in her treatise. She cannot imagine a cure for plague, and therefore cannot have her Blazing World practitioners imagine one when plague is an irregularity in nature. In other words, because plague is an irregularity of dissolving motions that normally produce natural decay in matter, the irregularity of the dissolving motion leads to an abnormal death. To the extent that it is abnormal, no scientist peering into nature will discern a pattern or its cause. It happens.

Although Cavendish has stated that there can be no cure, she has the Empress in her utopian fiction continue the interrogation of her Galenic physicians:

> The Empress being very desirous to know in what manner the plague was propagated and became so contagious, asked, whether it went actually out of one body into another? To which they answered, that it was a great dispute amongst the learned of the profession, whether it came by a division and composition of parts; that is, by expiration and inspiration; or whether it was caused by imitation: some experimental philosophers, said they, will make us believe, that by the help of their microscopes, they have observed the plague to be a body of little flies like atoms, which go out of one body into another, through the sensitive passages; the most experienced and wisest of our society, have rejected this opinion as a ridiculous fancy. (158–59)

The dispute related by the counselors is one Cavendish knew and understood personally, having embraced atomism early in her life and having replaced it in the end with something approximating vitalism. Here she displays her preferences, as "the most experienced and wisest" in the realm believe atomism is "a ridiculous fancy."

The key to understanding this debate is in *The Observations*:

> I have heard that a Gentleman in Italy fancied he had so good a Microscope, that he could see Atomes through it, and could also perceive the Plague; which he affirmed to be a swarm of

living Animals, as little as Atomes. . . . But . . . I do not believe
it to be a swarm of living Atomes flying up and down in the
Air; for if it were thus, then those Atoms would not remain in
one place, but infect all the places they passd through; when as
yet we observe, that the Plague will often be but in one Town
or City of a Kingdom, without spreading any further. . . . Since
it is often observed, that all Bodies are not infected, even in a
great Plague; it proves that the Infection is made by imitation;
and as one and the same Agent, cannot occasion the like effects in every Patient; as for example, Fire in several sorts of
Fuels; nay, in one and the same sort; as for example, in Wood;
for some wood takes sooner fire, and burns more clearly, and
dissolves more suddenly then some other; so it is also with the
Plague. (87–90)

Cavendish employs her own observations to refute the claim
of such atomists, supplying the reasoning behind the conclusions made by the Blazing World task force. We also begin
to see a trend here wherein Cavendish uses more fanciful
language in the description in her treatise than in her utopian
fiction. The "swarm of living Atoms flying up and down in
the Air" is quite a vivid picture after all, more vivid than
accounts from *The Blazing World*.

The Empress's practitioners conclude quite seriously that
"the most experienced and wisest of our land . . . do for the
most part believe, that [the plague] is caused by an imitation
of parts, so that the motions of some parts which are sound,
do imitate the motions of those that are infected, and that by
this means, the plague becomes contagious and spreading"
(159). In the estimation of the Blazing World Galenists, then,
plague appears as kin to that in Bacon's *The Natural History* —
an amorphous, elastic entity obeying the rules of similitude
alone. Yet never in her treatises of natural philosophy or in
The Blazing World does Cavendish consider bubonic plague
as emanating from odors, prisons, or infectious imaginations,
as Bacon does. She does not depict plague in elastic or figurative
form. Plague refers only to the particular disease, and this is

another point at which her writing on plague departs from that by others.

The practitioners' notion that an imitation of parts causes the plague calls to mind the Paracelsian model of disease, wherein an ill essence (*astrum*) of one being can corrupt the essence of another. In fact, the conclusion the Blazing World Galenists give is not at all Galenic, nor is it firm. They do not say that they themselves believe or have proven that this imitation occurs. They refer to others elsewhere who are wiser as those best able to judge, but they never tell us who these other wiser people are, and the Empress does not ask. Moreover, even those wise men believe "for the most part" but without unanimity or force. In the end, then, the Blazing World Galenists know nothing more than Cavendish does. She tells us more about what plague is not than what it is. Bubonic plague is not a bunch of atoms flying up and down. The atomic theory is ill-conceived, but perhaps more disconcerting, her Galenic practitioners find no alternative wholly convincing.

With regard to plague in utopia, we might easily determine that Cavendish was more restricted in her thinking than were her predecessors. To imagine a universal contagion with no cure is more confining than to imagine, like Thomas More and Francis Bacon, that a nation might fortify itself against plague by means of moderate behavior or scientific advancement. Cavendish does not expose the dangers of utopian projects, like Jonson and Shakespeare, but like them, she cannot offer much comfort in plague-time. In Cavendish's world, the plague is universally contagious, no longer within the lunulae of the earring; finding a cure for this plague is as likely as finding the mythical philosopher's stone.

We can, however, account for Cavendish's lack of prescription. Cavendish did not have a program for soul, for science, or for society. She had instead a program for her own imagination. Her lack of an established religious, scientific, or social program limited her ability to prescribe. As a case in point, her utopia is the only one that does not entertain the idea of quarantines: all others in this study — and every other work of literature grappling with bubonic plague at any length — do so in some form, but Cavendish does not.

On the other hand, lack of a program also freed her from that very script, allowing her to venture in new directions. With this freedom, Margaret Cavendish was able to move vast lengths in her thinking over time: from pondering humoral causes of things, to imagining vitalistic motions; from contemplating worlds isolated from or within other worlds to conceiving of connected globes and multiple, inhabited planets; and from imagining microcosmic worlds where people danced at balls to creating worlds where the inhabitants are mixed human-animal species. In these ways among others, Margaret Cavendish thought beyond the limits that other early modern utopists established for themselves. She thought toward what might be by building on the platforms available to others, aware of the best practices available, and then she played with them, squeezing them into almost unrecognizable and in many instances downright absurd forms. We cannot with ease place her amidst the likes of More and Bacon or Shakespeare and Jonson.

Cavendish was also exceptional with respect to her depictions of plague. In her writings, she poignantly stages her own struggle to understand the literal disease. She is also more rigorous in her merging of science and literature. To my knowledge, no other writer in England of her time or before left such extensively interrelated works. No other so carefully marks for us by repeated demonstration the boundaries — or lack thereof — between science and fiction, and no other provides us with so many angles — dramatic, poetic, and narrative, personal, scientific, and aesthetic — from which to assess the plague. In this, Cavendish initiated what would become an urge to move beyond utopia as a genre and into science fiction as we know it today.

EIGHT

Fables and Fancies

The Style of Hope in
Bacon and Cavendish

Seen side-by-side, the twin works of Francis Bacon and Margaret Cavendish have much in common. Each writer intentionally complements natural philosophy with a literary utopia. Each uses the utopia as a space of practice for his or her scientific observations, putting them into action before the readers' eyes. Each narrator appears to be reliable. We do not encounter a Surly, a Hythloday (potentially speaking nonsense), or even a Gonzalo, as sweet as he is. Instead the narrators tell us in a straightforward manner what they witnessed, and although Cavendish's narrator turns out to be the Duchess of Newcastle herself, and Bacon's seems convinced that Bensalemites are worthy of imitation, each includes enough detail to convince us that we are reading about a very human population, however unusual they may be.

By comparing the paired texts, we gain insight into each author's conception of the human condition. We also see the pairs — and their author's conceptions — as surprisingly less similar than we might have expected. In the preface to the *Blazing World*, Cavendish explains exactly how she sees the relationship between the more reasonable and the more fanciful texts she joined:

> If you wonder, that I join a work of fancy to my serious philosophical contemplations; think not that it is out of a disparagement to philosophy . . . [the latter] is a more profitable and useful study than this [of fancy], so it is also more laborious and difficult, and requires sometimes the help of fancy, to recreate the mind, and withdraw it from its more serious contemplations. And this is the reason, why I added this piece of fancy to my philosophical observations, and joined them as two worlds at the ends of their poles. . . . But lest my fancy should stray too much, I chose such a fiction as would be agreeable to the subject treated of in the former parts.[1]

The Blazing World depends upon its scientific precursor, which in turn depends upon it. As worlds joined at their poles, they are scales balanced against each other, each necessary for accurate measure of the other.

It is possible that Cavendish borrowed from the works of Francis Bacon, using his paired texts as a model. But we have absolutely no evidence to support this hypothesis — no evidence supplied by a woman who enjoyed naming those natural philosophers whose works she thought more arrogant than learned. Bacon would have been among them. In any case, Cavendish followed Bacon, intentionally or not, in the old trick of scientists as defined by Lucretius in *De Rerum Natura* — a work that Robert Schuler in *Francis Bacon and Scientific Poetry* has termed "the single most important and influential scientific poem of antiquity."[2] Lucretius explains his prescription for education:

As with children, when physicians try to administer rank wormwood, they first touch the rims about the cups with the sweet yellow fluid of honey, that unthinking childhood be deluded as far as the lips, and meanwhile may drink up the bitter juice of wormwood, and though beguiled be not betrayed, but rather by such means be restored and regain health, so now do I . . . if by chance in such a way I might engage your mind in my verses, while you are learning to see in what shape is framed the whole nature of things.[3]

Bacon and Cavendish knew that to move an audience, you must bring more than raw truth into view; you must appeal to the senses. In this regard, as they positioned the language of science within more engaging contexts, Bacon and Cavendish have much in common.

Students of Bacon's *New Atlantis* have examined his paired texts, concluding that his science and fiction together provide the best picture of his entire program for natural philosophy. Among many, Rose-Mary Sargent writes that the *New Atlantis* provided "a concrete plan for the establishment of a scientific society";[4] Denise Albanese also sees the *New Atlantis* as a means for furthering Bacon's scientific and specifically utopian agenda.[5] These observations are now common among those studying *New Atlantis*. Many critics have also assessed the poetic qualities of the language Bacon chose for his scientific works. Robert M. Schuler and John Channing Briggs discuss Bacon's display of an unresolved tension between science and poetry, between reason and imagination, truth and myth.[6]

The same might be done for Cavendish. In *Margaret Cavendish and the Exiles of the Mind*, Anna Battigelli confirms, "Readers tend to read *Observations* and *Blazing World* separately, but the two are in fact companion pieces; although the former takes the form of the scientific discourse and the latter of romantic fantasy, both are philosophical texts aimed at contesting the Royal Society's experimental program by specifically targeting Hooke's celebration of microscopes and telescopes."[7] She does not examine Cavendish's science in order to comment further upon it or upon its place in the utopian writing. Nevertheless, Battigelli is more attentive to Cavendish's legitimate scientific endeavors than many who view Cavendish as writing and thinking within a vacuum.

Collette V. Michael concludes, "By today's standards, much of what Margaret wrote is erroneous, but there is a candor and naiveté that retains its freshness and point of view not corrupted by the 'official' teachings of the time."[8] The problems with this view are obvious to those studying Cavendish within the context of early modern scientific history. Cavendish's views were indeed corrupted by the teachings of the time. Her early treatises on natural philosophy either parroted or struck out boldly against the "official" teachings of Bacon, Boyle, and Hobbes. She could not, at least initially, think about natural philosophy without thinking about those who came before her, from whose writings she learned. It took Cavendish years to develop a confident and independent assessment of natural philosophy, but even then, she was always aware of what others were espousing.

Determined to remove Cavendish from the vacuum created by scholars and to place her squarely within the seventeenth century of which she was a prominent and clearly popular part, John Rogers remains faithful to the language and concepts of the day when tracing the development in Cavendish's scientific treatises. Rogers then focuses on Cavendish's political position and her intention to inspire women in their thinking and writing.[9] Battigelli concludes similarly, "Cavendish was finally less interested in atomism as a theory of matter than as an explanatory discourse for the political and emotional turmoil that surrounded her" (39). Even when Cavendish shifted her views of the world from Atomistic to vitalistic, "her primary interest lay not in the nature of the physical universe but rather in the nature of the human mind."[10]

The problem with this interpretation is that natural philosophy and by extension the bubonic plague become all but inconsequential considerations, when in fact they were essential, built into her works repeatedly and overtly. Cavendish saw herself as someone thinking and writing about natural philosophy. Only secondarily did she realize that her gender might get in the way of her pursuing her primary goal. We see this if we turn to the works themselves, because she only raises the issue of her gender when she addresses the reader. In the works themselves, she attends to the business of natural philosophy, to which all else caters.

A fit companion for Francis Bacon in this regard, Cavendish saw fancy and reason "joined . . . as two worlds at the ends of their poles" (*Observations* 124). Bacon had seen his own pairing in nearly identical terms. Bacon had left *New Atlantis* incomplete and without a preface at his death in 1626. But one year later, his editor and chaplain William wrote the missing preface and published the paired works:

> This fable my Lord devised, to the end that he might exhibit therein a model or description of a college instituted for the interpreting of nature and the producing of great and marvelous works for the benefit of men, under the name of Salomon's House. . . . Certainly the model is more vast and high than can possibly be imitated in all things; notwithstanding most things therein are within men's power to effect.[11]

Rawley goes on to explain the reason that Bacon stopped short of completing the "fable" that was to include a group of laws for governing the commonwealth: "foreseeing it would be a long work, his [Bacon's] desire of collecting the *Natural History* diverted him, which he preferred many degrees before it. This work of the *New Atlantis* (as much as concerneth the English edition) his Lordship designed for this place; in regard it hath so near affinity (in one part of it) with the preceding *Natural History*" (3:127). By publishing the works together, Rawley formalized that affinity between the fictional *New Atlantis* and the scientific text of observation, *The Natural History*.

Bacon saw *The Natural History* as the foundation for his plan to advance human understanding and control of nature, so why not leave it standing alone? Why pair it with *New Atlantis*? Perhaps it was an accident. But more likely it was an intentional choice on the part of the man who understood Bacon's program and saw that the reception of the primary work might be made sweeter, in Lucretian terms, if fable went with it. It makes sense that a fictional realm showing the end result of a scientific program not yet begun would help sell the building blocks of the program. In any case, Rawley's decision, if it was only his and not also Bacon's, was right: the texts remained together through 14 additional publications within the century.[12]

It appears that Bacon and Cavendish had a common understanding of the relationship between fact and fiction, reality and imagination: "fancy" or "fable" and "serious philosophical contemplations" go hand in hand, complementing each other. Certainly for each of the authors, "fable" and "fancy" denote forms of thinking and writing that are different from and less important than the more reasonable counterparts of natural philosophy. Yet Bacon would never have applied the term "fancy" to his work. Bacon considered fancy to be the result of decayed reasoning. Poetry was one of its primary manifestations, "which," he writes in *De Augmentis*, "commonly exceeds the measure of nature, joining at pleasure things which in nature would never have come together, and introducing things which in nature would never have come to pass; just as Painting likewise does. This is the work of Imagination" (5:292). Moreover, poetry is "as a plant which comes from the lust of the earth without a formal seed, it has sprung up and spread abroad more than any kind of learning" (318). In this particularly misleading form of poetry, fancy hinders the advancement of learning. It keeps one trapped in a whirlpool of self-reflection with no anchor, no "formal seed."

How then does Bacon account for his own seemingly fanciful utopian text?[13] He calls it a "fable" in order to distinguish it from common poetry. In *De Augmentis*, he determines that "fable," however poetically rendered it may be, is a very special and ancient form of "parabolic" poetry:

> Religion itself commonly uses it [parabolic poetry] and as a means of communicating between divinity and humanity. . . . Now this method of teaching, used for illustration, was very much in use in the ancient times. For the inventions and conclusions of human reason (even those that are now common and trite) being then new and strange, the minds of men were hardly subtle enough to conceive them, unless they were brought nearer to the sense by this kind of resemblances and examples. And hence the ancient times are full of all kinds of fables, parables, enigmas, and similitudes. (5:317)

Fables and parables are the acceptable poetry because they are so ancient that they are untainted. They were practical media for delivery of divine truth to humans, what Bacon calls "natural divination" in the *New Atlantis* and elsewhere, including within the *Magnalia Naturae*.

By natural divination, human beings could make sense of nature, shaping it toward its divine ends as discerned through revelation. Natural divination in the form of fable or parable, might lead one along a path from right point to right point, closer and closer to truth, to God — never to the titillation of base poetry. Fables and parables were in fact the best modes for communicating such divinity, and Bacon took it upon himself to record with clarity some of those important parables in *De Augmentis*: "But since that which has hitherto been done in the interpretation of these parables, being the work of unskillful men, not learned beyond common places, does not by any means satisfy me, I think it fit to set down philosophy according to the Ancient Parables" (317–18). If recorded and read with care, Bacon's fables would serve as the building blocks of truth in the world, delivered through divination.

In this context, the *New Atlantis* perfectly complements *The Natural History* and all natural philosophy: fable is a bridge from the divine to human, which, in Bacon's words from the *History*, "takes off the mask and veil from natural objects, which are commonly concealed and obscured under the variety of shapes and external appearances" (5:257). Both the fable and the natural history operate similarly within Bacon's understanding of humankind's place in the universe. Humans were created to be above, separate from, and in control of nature. With the Fall, humans forgot their place, and their minds became enslaved to idols. In the postlapsarian cosmological system, "nature exists in three stages": "Either she is free, and develops herself in her own ordinary course; or she is forced out of her proper state by the perverseness and insubordination of matter and the violence of impediments, or she is constrained and moulded by art and human ministry" (5:253). Bacon determines to educate us toward the last stage, which, according to John Channing Briggs means, "The new sciences aspire to remake an Eden for human knowledge in tandem with Divinity's repair of man's moral condition."[14] In this program, fable functions to reintroduce readers to God and to the possibility of Edenic life on earth by helping them in turn to mould nature, starting with codification of its natural history.

Cavendish, on the other hand, saw such high-aspiring art as nothing more than hot air. By 1666, she could not allow her natural philosophy to speak for God, because she considered all beings (human, animal, stone, etc.) to be only part of the whole that was God. In other words, no single part of the whole could know the whole, let alone perceive any of the intentions or revelations of that whole in order to direct its own actions by them. Certainly, then, no one could claim to know God or the God-designed plan for controlling nature.

In addition to this, Nature had her own plan, as Cavendish relates in *Observations Upon Experimental Philosophy*: "Nature is but one body, it is intirely wise and knowing, ordering her self-moving parts with all facility and ease, without any disturbance, living in pleasure and delight, with infinite varieties and curiosities, such as no single Part or Creature of hers can ever attain to" (4). Within those "infinite varieties," Nature ultimately acts in a cyclical manner to the extent that the decay of one organism becomes the life-giving substance of another. Death is the beginning of life rather than a repercussion of Adam and Eve's Fall.[15]

In her mature writings, Cavendish rejects an atomistic, mechanical natural philosophy that views nature as unruly and in need of regulation by us: "Some are of opinion," she writes in *Observations Upon Experimental Philosophy*,

> That by Art there can be a reparation made of the Mischiefs and Imperfections mankind has drawn upon it self by negligence and intemperance, and a wilful and superstitious deserting the Prescripts and Rules of Nature, whereby every man, both from a derived Corruption, innate and born with him, and from his breeding and converse with men, is very subject to slip into all sorts of Errors. But the all-powerful God, and his servant Nature, know, that Art, which is but a particular Creature, cannot inform us of the Truth of the Infinite parts of Nature, being but finite itself. . . . Man is but a small part, and his powers are but particular actions of Nature, and therefore he cannot have a supreme and absolute power. (5–6)

Cavendish rejects the ultimate ends of Baconian natural philosophy, and, by extension, of Paracelsian theory, convinced that art cannot rectify nature.

"The truth is," she explains, "the more the figure by Art is magnified, the more it appears mis-shapen from the natural, in so much as each joynt will appear as a diseased, swell'd and tumid body, ready and ripe for incision" (9).[16] In this passage, Cavendish refers to the microscope but speaks of all such instruments of art — chemical or mechanical — that change our perception of nature. By her assessment, they can not help to perceive nature more accurately, and they certainly can not shape it toward divine ends.[17]

The problem is that — logical or entertaining by our standards or not — Cavendish's approach does not finally leave enough room for what we consider scientific experimentation and advancement. In respect to medical experimentation for example, Cavendish appears to take a passive position of resignation, stating in "Of the Universal Medicine, and of Diseases," "Nay, they might soon make or create a new Matter, then rectifie the irregularities of Nature more then Nature herself is pleased to do; for though Art may be an occasion of the changes of some parts or motions, of their compositions and divisions, imitations, and the like; like as a Painter takes a copy from an original, yet it cannot alter Infinite Nature" (80–81). With such declarations, Cavendish certainly removes herself from the circles of those doing what we might call legitimate science. Cavendish almost says, "Why bother trying out medicines when nature is unknowable?" In the case of curing disease, Cavendish turns a bit practical and admits to some benefit in experimentation toward remedy:

> To Return to the Universal Medicine; although I do not believe there is any, nor that all Diseases are curable; yet my advice is, that no applications of remedies should be neglected in any disease whatsoever; because Diseases cannot be so perfectly known, but that they may be mistaken; and so even the most experienced Physician may many times be deceived, and mistake a curable disease for an incurable; wherefore Trials should be made as long as life lasts. (82)

Cavendish walks a fine line. While nearly eliminating the active component of her philosophical program, she prescribes trials.

As for fancy, it fits with Cavendish's view of a cyclical and uncontrollable Nature within which the decay of one organism becomes the life-giving substance of another. One can no better compel the mind to be always reasonable than compel nature to heal herself. As humans need sleep in order to be productive, so do minds churning on the reasonable discourses of science need free time to play. As much as she feared its destructive power over lives when grown to excess, Cavendish appreciated decay and its many forms as a part of the human condition.

The difference between Baconian and Cavendishean natural philosophy is larger than conflict over politics, greater than gender, and it moves beyond the debates among mechanists, vitalists, atomists, monists, Galenists and Paracelsians. The only suitable arena for this debate is cosmological — a forum larger than that required for discussion of More and Bacon and a forum that from this time forward in the western world would never again shrink in size. Western utopianism and scientific inquiry would demand a cosmological view and would then only undergo increasing change. In the latter half of the seventeenth century, at the hands of Jonathan Swift and Joseph Hall utopia would prove laughable, while William Harvey and Thomas Sydenham would radically alter internal medicine and pave the way for epidemiology. By the early nineteenth century, utopia would prove deadly and demand renaming as dystopia.

NINE

The Rectification of Air and the Pursuit of Paradise

When plague visited England, from its first visitation until its last, people generally agreed that although God was its primary cause, the secondary cause was most often the air. The air could carry upon it pestiferous vapors harmful to the very life force of the body. In plague-time more than at any other, the air became suspect. We can also account for the extreme appreciation of pure air in this time by turning to Aristotle and the natural philosophers who followed him. They contended that the primary purpose for breathing was to keep the innate and life-giving heat of the body regulated.[1] Breathing in allowed cool air to prevent the innate heat of the body from growing beyond measure. Exhalation expelled the hot breath tainted with excess heat.[2] Foul the air, and you disrupt the respiration process.

In England, Thomas More, Francis Bacon, and Margaret Cavendish were among many who considered the best practices of the time as they imagined and wrote about regions where the air was pure and self-cleansing.[3] Shakespeare and Jonson were among many who captured plague-murdered hope in dramatic form. By the latter half of the seventeenth century, as the country began to recover from Civil War, increasing air pollution and continued threats from bubonic plague made it clear that England must continue to battle for its well being. Fortunately, many of England's most powerful minds were enlisted in the campaign. From the first study of pneumatics and advances in sanitation and quarantine practices to the literary efforts of John Milton and Margaret Cavendish, the seventeenth century saw a general preoccupation with the air, channeled into a concerted effort to understand and improve it.[4]

Extended at the national level, the reasons to fear a foul wind were clear. John Evelyn — a prominent royalist, keeper of the now-famous diary, and founding member of the Royal Society — confirms this in the first page of his open letter to Charles II and Parliament, titled *Fumifugium: or, The Inconveniencie of the Aer and Smoak of London Dissipated* (1661): "the Aer itself is many times a potent and great disposer to Rebellion" (1; see figure 9).[5] Although London's geographic position makes it naturally healthful, he explains, fumes from an increase in coal usage and the unsanitary practices of butchers have fouled the air, which might easily lead to another large-scale rebellion if not cleaned up.[6]

Given the many reasons for an early modern preoccupation with the air, it is not surprising to find both Cavendish and Milton writing about the subject in works that date from around the time of the Great Plague and fire of London. What is surprising is the degree of overlap in their major fictional narratives. Both Cavendish in *The Blazing World* and Milton in *Paradise Lost* discuss the fall of humankind, both create

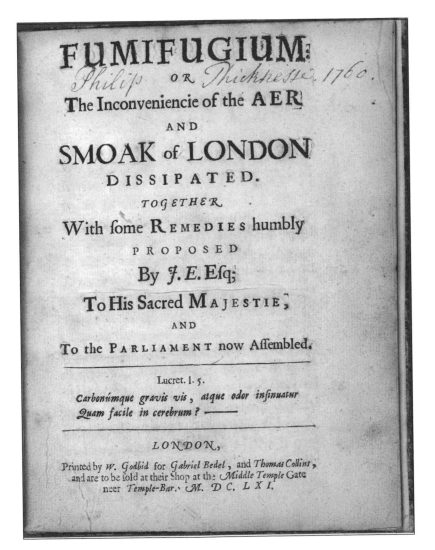

FUMIFUGIUM:

Philip OR *Thicknesse. 1760.*

The Inconveniencie of the AER

AND

SMOAK of LONDON

DISSIPATED.

TOGETHER

With some REMEDIES humbly

PROPOSED

By *J. E.* Esq;

To His Sacred MAJESTIE,

AND

To the PARLIAMENT now Assembled.

Lucret. l. 5.

Carbonúmque gravis vis, atque odor insinuatur
Quam facile in cerebrum? ———

LONDON,

Printed by *W. Godbid* for *Gabriel Bedel*, and *Thomas Collins*, and are to be sold at their Shop at the *Middle Temple* Gate neer *Temple-Bar.* *M. DC. LXI.*

Figure 9. From John Evelyn, *Fumifugium* (Wing E3489). Title page.
By permission of the Huntington Library.

angelic characters who educate humanity, both include humans who are exceptionally inquisitive with respect to the world around them, and both authors name their regions of pure air "Paradise." By examining the air within each narrative — its power to heal or to harm, and the power of humans to control it — we gain an understanding of how Cavendish and Milton conceive of the human condition.

Cavendish published the *Blazing World* after a lengthy stay in London and after the Great Plague visited the city. The tale begins with a young lady who, after a kidnapping gone awry, finds herself alone and headed toward the North Pole, with no way to control the vessel. She survives because her beauty, we are told, radiates a light that preserves her in those arctic temperatures. It rarefies the air. Traveling through the North Pole, the lady finds herself in another world connected to her own at its pole. There, creatures who are half fox or bear and half human discover the lady and ultimately decide that, due to her radiance, she is best suited to inhabit Paradise, the city of their Emperor. They travel by boat and, if we were not already impressed by those creatures who "showed her all civility and kindness imaginable" (127) and who spoke a common language whether they were bird-, fox-, bear-, worm-, or monkey-men, then we are impressed by the fact that the inhabitants of the Blazing World have very few enemies, and experience no war.

Their only enemies are threats from nature, and it seems that they have overcome the majority of these with technology, harnessing even the wind. As the bear- and fox-men escort the lady to the Emperor, they travel through the ocean at ease:

> They had an extraordinary art, much to be taken notice of by experimental philosophers, and that was a certain engine, which would draw in a quantity of air, and shoot forth wind with a great force; this engine in a calm, they placed behind their ships, and in a storm, before; for it served against the raging waves,

like canons against an hostile army, or besieged town. . . . Using two of those engines at every ship, one before to beat off the waves, and another behind to drive it on; so that the artificial wind had the better of the natural; for it had a greater advantage of the waves than the natural of the ships. (128–29)

Harness the air with such a machine and you govern the winds and the waves. From there, you can control the seas, and rule the world — a lesson that would not be lost on citizens of an island nation.

Upon meeting the lady, the Emperor makes her his Empress, and she reigns in Paradise, entertained by societies of chemists, mathematicians, Galenists, natural philosophers, spirits, and a companion for her soul, in the form of Margaret Cavendish, the Duchess of Newcastle herself. At some point, however, the lady determines to help her land of origin attain the peace she has in the Blazing World. In "The Second Part of the Description of the New Blazing World," the Empress applies her power over the air to win the war. In the last battle, the Empress commands her bird- and worm-men to destroy the homes of her motherland's enemies, telling them,

To lay some of the fire-stones at the bottom of those supporters [of the houses], and when the tide came in, all their houses were of a fire, which did so rarefy the water, that the tide was soon turned into vapor and this vapor again into air; which caused not only a destruction of their houses, but also a general barrenness over all their country that year, and forced them to submit as well as the rest of the world had done. Thus the Empress did not only save her native country, but made it the absolute monarch of that entire world. (214)

Like dropping a nuclear bomb, Cavendish's Empress alters the natural world, by making the air a bane to inhabitants.

She becomes the Prince of the Air, as it were, and stands unopposed in power, able to create or destroy other nations and worlds as she desires. In this way, she makes an interesting character for comparison with Milton's Satan in *Paradise Lost,* particularly given the fact that she is seen as a positive figure, healing the world from which she came. In celebrating victory, the Empress stages a pageant:

> The bird-men carried her upon their backs into the air, and there she appeared as glorious as the sun. Then she was set down upon the seas again, and presently there was heard the most melodious and sweetest consort of voices, as ever was heard out of the seas, which was made by the fish-men; this consort was answered by another, made by the bird-men in the air, so that it seemed as if sea and air had spoke and answered each other by way of singing dialogues, or after the manner of those plays that are acted by singing voices. (215)

She seems to command the sun, almost becoming it, able to draw up the vapors and dry the air for health or for harm, as she desires. With the light, heat, and air at her command, her own citizens will live in health and prosperity without fear of harm. What enemy will dare attack? And her people will be well entertained. What court pageant could ever have rivaled this show?

In contrast, when the Empress desires to visit the homeland of her soul's companion, the Duchess of Newcastle, she is warned that it is nothing like the Blazing World. The Duchess's England wastes away under a blanket of vapors, as she explains to the Empress: "The world you are going into, is dark at nights . . . and not so full of blazing-stars as this world is, which make as great a light in the absence of the sun, as the sun doth when it is present; for that world hath but little blinking stars, which make more shadows than light, and are only able to draw up vapors from the earth, but not to rarefy or clarify them, or to convert them into serene air" (207). While the Blazing World itself respires and digests in health, as its very name might suggest, England belches and is . . . windy. In the end, after a brief visit into the fumy world of her friend, the Empress chooses to stay in her Paradise, where it "is always clear, and never subject to any storms, tempests, fogs, or mists, but has only refreshing dews that nourish the earth; the air of it is sweet and temperate" (222). The kidnapped heroine of the romance has her happy ending. She rules in a land where the air is healthier than that in her land of origin or in England, and where she can command the winds whenever she needs extra protection or desires entertainment.

When we turn to *Paradise Lost*, first published only a year after *The Blazing World*, we find a subtler and more pervasive treatment of respiration, but the greatest threat to humans still comes on the air. In *Paradise Lost* every breath of life, every exhalation of foulness, every comet, every perfumed prayer, every inspiration, and every aspiration speaks of the importance of the respiratory process in creation and in destruction.[7] Milton begins with this last idea, taking his readers directly into the toxic exhalation of fiery hell, where all is smoke and stench, all the breeding place of plague. There we first find Satan, the Prince of the Air with whom we are familiar, lurching up from the fiery flood:

> on each hand the flames
> Driv'n backward slope thir pointing spires, and roll'd
> In billows, leave i' th' midst a horrid Vale.
> Then with expanded wings he steers his flight
> Aloft, incumbent on the dusky Air
> That felt unusual weight, till on dry Land
> He lights, if it were Land that ever burn'd
> With solid, as the Lake with liquid fire;
> And such appear'd in hue; as when the force
> Of subterranean wind transports a Hill
> Torn from *Pelorus*, or the shatter'd side
> Of thundring *Ætna*, whose combustible
> And fuell'd entrails thence conceiving fire,
> Sublim'd with Mineral fury, aid the Winds,

> And leave a singed bottom all involv'd
> With stench and smoke: Such resting found the sole
> Of unblest feet.[8]

Exhaled into hell, the rebellious, combustible crew of fallen angels find themselves in the equivalent of Evelyn's smoky London and the land of the Empress's enemies after the last battle. No life is sustained here where the stench and smoke cannot permit true respiration. The inner heat of the body will always burn too hot. The inhalation will in Hell never inspire. Hell — and, we can assume, Satan — will only belch pestilence-producing wind.

So, when Satan first experiences Paradise, he is inspired as much by the air as by the sight:

> And of pure now purer air
> Meets his approach, and to the heart inspires
> Vernal delight and joy, able to drive
> All sadness but despair: Now gentle gales
> Fanning their odoriferous wings dispense
> Native perfumes, and whisper whence they stole
> Those balmy spoils. As when to them who sail
> Beyond the *Cape of Hope,* and now are past
> Mozambic, off at Sea North-East winds blow
> Sabean odours from the spicy shore
> Of Araby the blest; with such delay
> Well pleas'd they slack thir course, and many a League
> Cheer'd with the grateful smell old Ocean smiles.
> So entertain'd those odorous sweets the fiend
> Who came thir bane.
>
> (4.153–67)

Here, Satan comes to Paradise as bane to the sweetness that mingles in the air. According to this simile of the sailors, Eden should renew hope with just one whiff. The scent does not work well enough on Satan's corrupted mind. Although the inhalation of Paradise inspires Satan to reverie, his desire to exhale his own pestiferous breathe upon the air is stronger.

But before he contaminates the environment, Satan takes one last snuff of a pure and potentially rectifying Paradise. He sees — or perhaps we should say, he smells — Eve, whom he finds alone for the first time:

> *Eve* separate he spies,
> Veild in a Cloud of Fragrance, where she stood,
> Half spi'd, so thick the Roses bushing round
> About her glow'd . . .
>
> . . . .
>
> Much hee the Place admir'd, the Person more.
> As one who long in populous City pent,
> Where Houses thick and Sewers annoy the Air,
> Forth issuing on a Summer's Morn to breathe
> Among the pleasant Villages and Farmes
> Adjoyn'd, from each thing met conceives delight,
> The smell of Grain, or tedded Grass, or Kine,
> Or Dairie, each rural sight, each rural sound;
> If chance with Nymphlike step fair Virgin pass,
> What pleasing seem'd, for her now pleases more,
> She most, and in her look sums all Delight.
>
> (9.424–54)

One can imagine the Londoner who, pent within the populous city, emerges into the fresh air of the countryside. Particularly in plague-time, the country air would seem a panacea in itself, even without the added bonus of the virgin. In miniature this is how the air adorning Eve might affect us. One whiff and we would be rejuvenated. But Satan's corruption is too great for this remedy, and the simile suggests that his determination to pollute the pure air of Eden and to taint the ambrosial fragrance of Eve is entirely unnatural and reprehensible.

For a time, Satan succeeds in his efforts, polluting the air and the minds in Paradise. He begins by tempting Eve through dream to reconsider her Edenic environment. Afterwards, as she explains to Adam, "One shap'd and wing'd like one of those from Heav'n" led her to the tree of knowledge (5.55). There the seeming angel encouraged her to taste of its fruit by first conjuring an image of flight:

> Taste this, and be henceforth among the Gods
> Thyself a Goddess, not to Earth confin'd,
> But sometimes in the Air, as wee, sometimes
> Ascend to Heav'n, by merit thine, and see
> What life the Gods live there, and such live thou.
>
> (5.78–81)

In the dream the disguised Satan offers Eve a bite of the fruit, and with the smell alone — for we do not know whether or not she tastes in the dream — she is transported:

> Forthwith up to the Clouds
> With him I flew, and underneath beheld
> The Earth outstretcht immense, a prospect wide
> And various: wond'ring at my flight and change
> To this high exaltation.
>
> (5.86–90)

Transported, Eve flies with Satan. In dream she is like Cavendish's Empress, a ruler of the air. The Empress's flights, however, do not cause her to question her role within the Blazing World. The Empress's flights instead enhance what she and her subjects already possess, and those flights are entirely within her control. Eve flies literally higher than the Empress — just far enough above Earth to permit her to taste the rarefied air from a region more sublime than Eden. Moreover, her flight is not freely tasted but one dependent upon Satan who alone determines flight time and altitude. While Cavendish's Empress secures greater freedom through flight, flight — or perhaps the scent preceding it — initiates Eve's loss of freedom.

It is not long after that that Satan stages the literal deception in much the same fashion. Of course, when Eve consumes the literal fruit, she does not ascend. Her falsely placed hope is exposed as fraud, but it is too late. After Adam joins her in the eating of the apple, the pair together fall into vaporous regions. Adam's view of Eve confirms the fall, as he proclaims,

> Never did thy Beauty since the day
> I saw thee first and wedded thee, adorn'd
> With all perfections, so enflame my sense
> With ardor to enjoy thee, fairer now
> Then ever, bountie of this virtuous Tree.
> So said he, and forbore not glance or toy
> Of amorous intent, well understood
> Of *Eve*, whose Eye darted contagious fire.
>
> (9.1028–036)

This contagious fire of passion will prove a conflagration when Adam and Eve realize that they have succumbed to their own literally hot desires.

They are tortured more internally than externally:

> Nor onely Tears
> Rain'd at thir Eyes, but high Winds worse within
> Began to rise, high Passions, Anger, Hate,
> Mistrust, Suspicion, Discord, and shook sore
> Thir inward State of Mind, calm Region once
> And full of Peace, now toss't and turbulent.
>
> (9.1121–126)

With "thir inward State of Mind" parched from the flames of passion and with the winds whipping up the passions, Adam and Eve are one step away from Evelyn's rebellion. Reason and Peace cannot live in such conditions.

Likewise, God cannot permit Adam and Eve to live in a pure realm, when their breaths might contaminate it.[9] God punishes them by literally putting them in their place — one outside of Eden, as if they were Eden's undigested waste. By altering the configuration of the earth and sun, God makes it impossible for the sun to draw up and dry the vapors as efficiently as it once had, just as Adam's reason can no longer rectify his emotions. The earth becomes ripe for imbalance of the elements, and thus plague on earth is born: "These changes in the Heav'ns, though slow, produc'd Like change on Sea and Land, sidereal blast, / Vapour, and Mist, and Exhalation hot, / Corrupt and Pestilent" (10.692–95). What follows this macrocosmic trauma is a microcosmic rebellion against it to the point of ushering in death, as beasts divide into hunter and prey (710–11).[10]

Soon human with human, and even human with himself, will fight, as Adam shortly thereafter reveals:

> O Conscience, into what Abyss of fears
> And horrors hast thou driv'n me; out of which
> I find no way, from deep to deeper plung'd!
> Thus *Adam* to himself lamented loud
> Through the still Night, not now, as ere man fell,
> Wholesome and cool, and mild, but with black Air
> Accompanied, with damps and dreadful gloom,
> Which to his evil Conscience represented
> All things with double terror.
>
> (10.842–49)

Plunged into the abyss, removed from the purifying light, Adam's mind, as Satan's, revolves in rebellion against humanity, against the very breath of life, against God: "Did I request thee, Maker, from my clay / To mold me Man?" (743–44). The breath of life within Adam seems to issue forth only pestilent vapor, contagious and deadly as Adam desires a death of the body and reveals the blow of despair, deadly to the soul, the ultimate punishment for turning traitor to one's master.

Fortunately (as Milton might want us to say) Adam and Eve realize that "the pure breath of Life, the Spirit of Man / Which God inspir'd" (784–85) still resides within them. Satan has become a bane to the air of Paradise, but he has not entirely extinguished their inspired breaths. As an outward sign of Adam and Eve's realization, "thir sighs the Air / Frequenting, sent from hearts contrite" (11.2–3) go forth, and those "sighs now breath'd/ Unutterable . . . the Spirit of prayer / Inspir'd, and wing'd for Heav'n" (11.5–7). In heaven, the sighs appear as prayers "clad / With incense" (17–18) and are named "first fruits" (22) by the Son of God. The Son then calls God's attention to those fruits of Adam and Eve, saying, "Accept me, and in mee from these [Adam and Eve] receive / The smell of peace toward Mankind" (37–38).[11] Adam and Eve's correct recognition of their place in the world first appears as a sigh that the Son perfumes for a more appealing presentation to God. God finds their labors acceptable.

For Milton's reader, these prayers take on a nearly tangible quality because of their scent. They also recall their opposite: the odor of carnage inhaled by and inspiring to Sin and Death, who are making plans to follow Satan to the now tainted Eden. Once God changes the constitution of the earth and creatures begin to hunt each other, Death,

> With delight he snuff'd the smell
> Of mortal change on Earth. As when a flock
> Of ravenous Fowl, though many a League remote,
> Against the day of Battle, to a field,
> Where Armies lie encampt, come flying, lur'd
> With scent of living Carcasses design'd
> For death, the following day, in bloody fight.
> So scented the grim Feature, and upturn'd
> His Nostril wide into the murky Air,
> Sagacious of his Quarry from so far.
>
> (10.272–81)

The battle lines are drawn. Sin and Death will hunt humans while the Son will help those who seek his intervention to cover that stench of mortality with perfumed and ultimately prophylactic prayers.

More than 50 years earlier, Lancelot Andrewes drew from the book of Revelation in order to recommended prayerful, perfumed protection in *A sermon of the pestilence Preached at Chiswick, 1603*:

> As the *Aire* is infected with *noisome sents* or *smels,* so the
> *infection* is removed by *sweet odours,* or *incense:* which *Aaron*
> did in the *Plague (put sweet odours in his Censer, and went*
> *betweene the living and the dead).* Now there is a fit
> resemblance between *Incense* and *Prayers: Let my prayer come*
> *before thy presence, as the Incense.* And when the *Priest* was
> within, burning Incense, *the people were without at their*
> *prayers.* And it is expressly said *that the sweet odours were*
> *nothing else but the prayers of the Saints.*[12]

England's plague orders, dating from 1578, had made it clear
year after year that the first step in plague prevention was to
create a "preservative by correcting the aire in Houses."[13]
Andrewes and Milton add to this preservative their own
perfumed prayers.

The notion of a battle over the air provided a sense of
control — particularly in plague-time. It allowed people to
believe that if they could alter the air, they might alter the
course of their lives. Some practiced what Andrewes and
Milton proposed by praying. Others attempted to harness the
air through technology like the inhabitants of the Cavendish's
Blazing World. Still others purchased amulets and watched
for comets and earthquakes and invented air purifiers of their
own — all in some fashion attempting to rectify the air.[14]

Of course, these efforts proved futile, and in retrospect they
seem rather laughable — that is, until we turn on our own
televisions sets and computers. For example, according to a
report in the *Chicago Tribune,* from April 2003:

> In Guangdong during the height of the SARS outbreak in Feb-
> ruary, the price of vinegar shot up to $12 a bottle from 60 cents
> as housewives kept pots of vinegar boiling on the kitchen stove
> in an effort to kill SARS germs. They also drank soup bowls of
> *ban lan gen,* a southern Chinese root. The *Beijing Evening News*
> laughed at both the vinegar and root soup stories, saying those
> remedies would not help. "But if you burn sandalwood and

Tibetan incense," the newspaper said, "it will have more effect." The paper also recommended keeping rooms well ventilated, being careful with pets and disinfecting elevators. But it failed to mention the first admonition of Western doctors: washing hands frequently.[15]

Many living in the infected regions of China believed on some level that the air had turned against them.[16] In recent years, we have also seen the equivalent of the plague doctor's uniform in the biohazard suits of officials trying to clean up after anthrax letters; we have read directions for the creation of safe rooms in our own homes; we have been encouraged to buy duct tape and plastic to seal our doors and windows against airborne terrorist agents; and we have seen men and women in the armed services outfitted against biological and chemical attack. The images alone cause us to reconsider the air.

Conclusion

When we do reconsider the air, we discover at least one obvious fact. We are not currently living in plague-time. Even when governments elevate national threat levels, we are many removes from the experiences of Thomas More, William Shakespeare, Ben Jonson, Margaret Cavendish, Francis Bacon, and John Milton. Although we may occasionally hear of temperatures above normal that kill hundreds, as in France during the summer of 2003, we do not worry that atmospheric change in an unusually hot summer will kill our loved ones. Although we fear for our troops abroad when they conduct operations in lands where biological or chemical weapons are thought to exist, we do not own manuals of instruction for cleansing the air in our homes. In partnership with the Centers for Disease Control and Prevention in the United States, the Department of Health in the United Kingdom, and Health Canada, the World Health Organization determines quarantine policies when necessary, but none of us can recite those policies, and none of us would challenge them if we became one of the individuals to whom they apply. We are safely beyond the plague-time of the past. We dwell in Davies's "no place," where our heads of state can safely rest.[1]

But we find ourselves here in part because people like King Henry VIII, Thomas More, Queen Elizabeth I, and Francis

Bacon planted seeds of utopia in plague-time — some more intentionally than others. They all practiced upon the platforms that were available to them and determined which would sustain the best practices for improving health. Natural philosophy and crowd control were clearly the most stable for several reasons. Perhaps most important, these platforms came to overlap, enforcing and enhancing the best practices of the other. For example, Queen Elizabeth's plague orders "executed throughout the Counties of this Realme" in 1578 and repeatedly thereafter contained within them a set of measures to control crowds. Always appended to them was medical "Advise set downe upon her Majesties expresse commandement, by the best learned in Physicke within this Realm." James I inherited and published these paired practices, and he passed them on as well. With each reign, they were slightly improved, growing to include Queen Anne's Quarantine Acts, which served as the basis for action in the cholera outbreak of the 1830s. Such plague orders, combining crowd control and natural philosophy, were never entirely retired, because they worked. Ultimately an evolutionary process, this passing on of best practices built us into the healthier present we currently experience.

Although the understanding of disease changed radically with the discovery of bacteria and of antibiotics at the end of the nineteenth century, the best practices for controlling plague are still those founded on the platforms of natural philosophy, which we now call science, and crowd control. The World Health Organization (WHO), The Centers for Disease Control and Prevention (CDC), The Department of Health (DOH), and Health Canada (HC) each have pages devoted to the bubonic plague, and each are government-funded science organizations.[2] When scientists employed by these organizations determine that it is in the public interest to restrict movement of populations, they turn to the governments involved in order to enforce their recommendations. Governments comply, and this should conjure up the image of Francis Bacon's Bensalemites, whose Minister of Health is an essential and powerful protector of the island.

These current organizations have produced webpages on bubonic plague. Admittedly, this publicized information serves primarily to satisfy citizen interest and to allay any concerns more than to disseminate timely instructions. However, there have been human outbreaks of bubonic plague, as the CDC reports: "In recent years, human plague has been reported in Africa from Angola, Botswana, Democratic Republic of the Congo, Kenya, Libya, Madagascar, Malawi, Mozambique, South Africa, Tanzania, Uganda, Zambia, and Zimbabwe; in Asia from Burma, China, India, Kazakhstan, Laos, Mongolia, and Vietnam; and in the Americas from Bolivia, Brazil, Ecuador, Peru, and the United States."[3] And it is only by actively monitoring bubonic plague that agencies can keep the disease bound within parentheses, as it were. In these ways, we build in the fashion of More's Utopians, Bacon's Bensalemites, and Cavendish's natural philosophers. We use science to serve government and government to serve science.

Like them, we have also determined that in the effort to create a better future on earth, the platform of religion will at best serve to reign in our zeal or, like a parent, to give us shelter from present pain. Religion will challenge us to be humble as we employ the best practices of science and crowd control, and it will suggest to us that we cannot improve our futures by human means alone. At worst, it will impede our progress, as it did hundreds of years ago in denying flight as a method of plague prevention. This realization came early and even to men like Thomas More, who, as we know, could not have displayed a greater devotion to the church than by giving his life. More did not condemn his pagan Utopians, and he does not allow the reader to do so, at least not with ease. In this way, by creating the literary utopia, Thomas More initiated the modern utopianism that we have inherited.

We have also inherited a secular form of the cautionary tale. By staging characters like Sir Mammon Epicure, Subtle, Timon, and Eve, the writers Ben Jonson, William Shakespeare, and John Milton reminded England that not all hope is stable. Sometimes false hope comes disguised as a new imaginary world promising health but delivering disease. This is true. If we are diagnosed with an incurable form of cancer, we would be wise to consider how many thousands of dollars we should spend on health retreats in foreign countries. On a more mundane level, the hope that causes millions of people to invest in lottery tickets may only increase the lack in their lives that initiated that hope. In such cases, we are reminded to build into our future with the knowledge that labor is required.

We do not inhabit plague-time with Thomas More, William Shakespeare, Ben Jonson, Francis Bacon, Margaret Cavendish, and John Milton. We never will — quite. We will never believe that the natural air will suddenly turn pestiferous. But we do believe — and should fear — that the natural air will be used against us by one of us. If this were the case, plague would likely come on the air as an aerosol — a breathable form of a lethal germ, one that Timon as *Misanthropos* would have paid dearly to possess. The consequences would be even more horrifying and all the more tragic. We do not inhabit plague-time with More, Shakespeare, Jonson, Bacon, Cavendish, and Milton. Yet their literary manifestations of utopianism succeed in warning us to be mindful of our air, to breathe freely, safely, and without fear, when we can. They encourage us to hope, while, for us, there is far more room to do so. They encourage us to harness that hope, steadfastly and creatively utilizing the best practices available. As we build into the future, they encourage us to challenge the limits within which we labor.

Notes

Notes to Introduction

1. There are other years when plague visited and caused distress, but these are the most prominent with respect to recorded deaths and the closing of Parliament. I have compiled these dates from a number of sources, especially from Paul Slack's *The Impact of Plague in Tudor and Stuart England*, 146–47. All future citations of this work will refer to page numbers in the text. I have compared Slack's dates with many sources, and those recording the years when the king or queen changed the Court term due to plague's presence in London are particularly helpful: see Charles Creighton, *History of Epidemics in Britain: From AD664 to the Extinction of the Plague*, 2 vols. 1:229–303; Charles Mullett, *The Bubonic Plague and England: An Essay in the History of Preventative Medicine*, 31–210. See also the *Short Title Catalogue* listings under "England, Proclamations": 1560, 1563, 1575–1578, 1604–1609, 1625, 1636. It is interesting to add the following visitations to the head of the list: Henry VI (1422–1461) 1433, 1449, 1451, 1454, 1457–1459; Edward IV (1461–1483) 1466–1467, 1471, and 1473.

2. Daniel Defoe, *A Journal of the Plague Year*, edited by Paula R. Backscheider, 156. All future citations of this work will refer to pages from this edition.

3. John Davies, *Humours heau'n on earth with the ciuile warres of death and fortune. As also the triumph of death: or, the picture of the plague, according to the life; as it was in anno Domini 1603* (1609), 233. All references to this poem will refer to page numbers from this edition.

4. Barbara Fass Leavy, *To Blight with Plague: Studies in a Literary Theme*; Margaret Healy, *Fictions of Disease in Early Modern England: Bodies, Plagues, and Politics*; Byron Lee Grigsby, *Pestilence in Medieval and Early Modern English Literature*.

5. Plague is all but absent from early modern biographies dating from before 1980, and we can account for the increase in interest in bubonic plague by noting that scholars were simultaneously studying AIDS as a modern plague and utilizing the critical approach of new historicism. Prior to this, biographies were often what we would now consider literary biographies or intellectual biographies rather than accounts of a life lived within certain times and places.

6. J. Leeds Barroll, *Politics, Plague and Shakespeare's Theater: The Stuart Years*, 4. All future citations of this work will refer to page numbers in the text.

7. Katherine Duncan-Jones, *Ungentle Shakespeare: Scenes from his Life*, 54. All future citations of this work will refer to page numbers in the text.

8. For a definition of the same terms in their early modern context, see especially Lancelot Andrewes, *A Sermon of the Pestilence Preached at Chiswick, 1603* (1636), 4. Hereafter cited in the text. Renaissance preachers often employed the following Old Testament references to plague in their sermons, confirming that the disease was a primary manifestation of God's wrath (these particular numbers refer to the King James version): Genesis 12.17; Exodus 9.14, 10.14; Numbers 11.33, 14,37, 16.46; Deuteronomy 28.58–59; Ps. 91.9–11, 106.28–31; Jeremiah 19.8, 49.17, 50.13; Hosea 13.14; Zechariah 14.12–18.

9. On Marco Polo's knowledge of Mandeville, see M. C. Seymour, introduction to *Mandeville's Travels*, John Mandeville, x.

10. John Mandeville, *Mandeville's Travels*, edited by M. C. Seymour, 211–12. All future citations of this work will refer to page numbers in the text.

11. Norman Cantor, *In the Wake of Plague: Black Death and the World it Made*. Every measure by which we gauge our lives — from our relationships to nature, our interactions with other human beings, and the way we govern ourselves, to the substance of our religions and our understanding of the role of art — each measure shifted in the "the wake of the plague." Cantor and others have suggested that with the decrease in population following plague came greater employment opportunities and avenues for challenging preexisting establishments. One might even ask, along with Cantor, "Did biomedical trauma then somehow trigger the Italian Renaissance?" (210). After all, we know plague directly touched the lives of Boccaccio and Petrarch when their loved ones died. It certainly compelled people — like Thomas More — to imagine change. In *Black Death and the Transformation of the West*, David Herlihy examines the population change brought about by the plague in 1348 and then discusses the resulting social and cultural effects, including

those we can see in art and literature. See also David Steel, "Plague Writing from Boccaccio to Camus": "There is a sense in which the age of modern fictions was ushered in by a virus" (90).

12. Elizabeth McCutcheon. "William Bullein's Dialogue Against the Fever Pestilence: A Sixteenth-Century Anatomy," in *Miscellanea Moreana: Essays for Germain Marc'hadour*, edited by Clare M. Murphy, Henri Gibaud, and Mario A. DiCesare, 343. Thanks to Lyman Tower Sargent for directing me to McCutcheon.

13. William Bullein's *A dialogue bothe pleasaunt and pietifull, wherein is a godlie regiment against the feuer pestilence with a consolation and comforte againste death* is here quoted from the 1888 Early English Text Society publication, *A Dialogue Against the Fever Pestilence*, edited by Mark W. Bullen and A. H. Bullen, Early English Text Society, 106. Although William Bullein added the utopian portion for the 1574 edition, the text edited by Bullen and Bullen is the 1578 version. Later in this examination, I will be referring to the original from 1564, which lacks the tale of Taerg Natrib and Nodnol. This will be indicated in the text by the date and in the notes.

14. Francis Bacon, *New Atlantis*, in *The Works of Francis Bacon*, edited by James Spedding, Robert L. Ellis, and Douglas D. Heath, 14 vols., 3.152. All following references to Bacon are from the Spedding volumes and will be cited in the text by volume and page number.

15. On Francis Bacon and the Royal Society, see Lyman Tower Sargent, "Utopian Traditions: Themes and Variations," in *Utopia: the Search for the Ideal Society in the Western World*, edited by Roland Schaer, Gregory Claeys, and Lyman Tower Sargent, 11.

16. Abraham Cowley quoted in Thomas Spratt, *The History of the Royal-Society of London* (1667).

17. For Sargent's definition of utopia, as well as his systematic approach to discussing dystopia, critical utopia, utopian satire, anti-utopia and utopianism, see Lyman Tower Sargent, "The Three Faces of Utopianism Revisited," 1–37. For further discussion of Sargent's apt terminology, see "Utopian Traditions: Themes and Variations" in *Utopia*, Schaer, Claeys, and Sargent, 8–15 and *The Utopia Reader*, edited by Gregory Claeys and Lyman Tower Sargent. Ben Jonson's *The Alchemist* and Shakespeare's *Timon of Athens*, for example, each have elements of utopian satire and of the anti-utopia, where the former is "a utopia that the author intended a contemporaneous reader to view as a criticism of the existing society" and as the latter is "a utopia that the author intended a contemporaneous reader to view as a criticism of utopianism or of some particular eutopia" (*Utopia Reader*, 2).

18. For those studying utopia, Bloch's three-volume study sets him on par with Thomas More. While Thomas More created the genre, Bloch most meticulously, usefully, and fruitfully examines it.

See Ernst Bloch, *The Principle of Hope*, 3 vols. Hereafter, Bloch is cited in text by volume and page number.

19. In "The Ones Who Walk Away From Omelas," Ursula K. Le Guin shows us this question embodied. Omelas is a society of order and beauty whose good depends on the suffering of one starved, filthy, abnormal child kept in a cellar. Those who cannot agree to the Faustian bargain do not gain initiation into the adulthood of peace in Omelas. They are the ones who walk away. They are the ones for whom the suffering in utopia exceeds its limits, for whom the utopia becomes dystopia, with flight the only recourse. For a broader discussion of Le Guin's short story, refer to *Utopian Studies* 2.1–2 (1991), which includes the story itself and a group of essays devoted to its examination.

20. Those interested in a side-by-side comparison of utopian works from France, Germany, and Italy should turn to Miriam Eliav-Feldon's *Realistic Utopias: the Ideal Imaginary Societies of the Renaissance 1516–1630*, Oxford Historical Monographs. My largest problem with Eliav-Feldon's study is her claim, "Utopia is a static society that has not evolved gradually but was created by fiat *ex nihilo*, has not changed since its creation, and is not destined to change in the future, since any change means deviation from perfection and therefore corruption. It is also a society artificially cut off from the course of human history. The utopias of the Renaissance in no way express a belief in the future, but at the same time they are no longer a lamentation of the past. All the utopias that are the subject of this study are described as existing or as possible in the present" (6). I disagree; however, Eliav-Feldon supplies useful descriptions of each utopian work, including a section on health.

21. For a discussion of early modern English utopian literature grounded in postmodern criticism, see Marina Leslie, *Renaissance Utopias and the Problem of History*. In short, Leslie argues that "Utopia in the sixteenth and seventeenth centuries . . . is best understood not as a self-reflexive retreat from history or a self-annihilating exposure of it but as a critical practice investigating the historical subject in the interrogative mode. I begin with the premise that utopian fictions . . . dramatize historical crisis" (8). Leslie does not examine cultural crisis, such as that created by plague. She instead focuses on the crisis of understanding history, a crisis that is predominantly intellectual and political.

22. This is a conservative estimate of the possible range for the play's creation, but some place it as early as 1604 and as late as 1613. With no evidence for the play's performance, some also suggest it never made it to the stage. On the subject of the plague visitation and the dating of *Timon*, see A. L. Rowse, *William Shakespeare: A Biography*, 416; F. P. Wilson, *The Plague in Shakespeare's London*, 119–20; Honan, *Shakespeare: A Life*, 347–49; and Barroll, 207.

23. For discussion of Harrington and Winstanley within the context of seventeenth century politics and utopia, see Robert Appelbaum, *Literature and Utopian Politics in Seventeenth-Century England.*

24. See John Bruce, "Milton's Mephitic Muse: Plague, Religion and the Infection Metaphor of *Paradise Lost,*" 238–48. Bruce stands alone in Milton scholarship, having published an exhaustive search throughout *Paradise Lost* for plague imagery. The problem is his zealous yet ultimately superficial treatment of the subject. Bruce fails to acknowledge the cultural understanding of disease with respect to Galenic and Paracelsian underpinnings. Without grounding his study in such data, Bruce's approach fails to satisfy scholars and may have only helped some of his readers to determine that assessing plague within the text is not a worthwhile venture. There are others whose scholarly work warrants consideration of plague; among them is Karen L. Edwards, whose chapter, "The Balm of Life" would benefit from a consideration of plague (in *Milton and the Natural World: Science and Poetry in Paradise Lost,* 182–98).

Notes to Chapter One

1. As noted by Robert Pollitzer, bubo distribution according to occurrence at prominent glandular regions is as follows: Groin 55–70 percent; Axillary (armpit) 20 percent; cervical (neck) or submaxillary (lower jaw) 10 percent (*Plague,* 420). All references to Pollitzer are from this edition and are cited by page number. Advanced stages of bubonic plague, the pneumatic and septicemic forms, kill nearly 100 percent of those who contract them. The primary characteristics of plague presented here are listed by each of the following: Paul Slack, 7–9 (see introduction, n. 1); Pollitzer, 418; Norman Cantor, 12–13 (introduction, n. 11); Carlo Cipolla, *Fighting the Plague in Seventeenth-Century Italy,* 104. Arlo Karlen converts the statistics on the septicemic form of plague into the language of experience: "People might get up healthy in the morning and die before night, raving and vomiting blood" (*Man and Microbe: Disease and Plagues in History and Modern Times,* 89).

2. Shrewsbury, J. F. D. *A History of Bubonic Plague in the British Isles,* 4–5. Records of physical symptoms from early modern texts match symptoms recorded in India and China in the twentieth century. See also Pollitzer (422) who verifies Shrewsbury's account.

3. The OED defines a botch as "a hump, swelling, a tumour, wen, or goiter." It was often used in place of "bubo," as can be seen in some of the primary sources cited. The term "botch" was used for "bubo" as early as 1338 in translations of the Bible by Wyclif, for

Deuteronomy 28.27: "The Lord shall smite thee with the botch of Egypt" [King James version]. The plague of 1348 had not yet occurred when Wyclif was writing, but later, readers would interpret Wyclif's "botch" as a plague-bubo.

4. John Taylor, *The fearefull summer, or, Londons calamity, the countries courtesy, and both their misery* (1625), A8. Taylor's poem was reprinted during the next major visitation in 1636. All references to this poem will include page numbers and letters to this 1625 edition.

5. Ambrose Paré, *The workes of that famous chirurgion Ambrose Parey translated out of Latine and compared with the French by Th: Johnson* (London, 1634), 831. All citations from this treatise will refer to pages from this edition. For more on Paré, see Nancy G. Siraisi, *Medieval and Early Renaissance Medicine: An Introduction to Knowledge and Practice*, 172, 186, 192.

6. Pollitzer, 207; see also 411–18. Serious attacks of plague in any form also commonly lead to abortion or miscarriage in pregnant patients (418).

7. John Caius, famed English Renaissance physician to Edward, Mary, and Elizabeth, discusses the difference between plague and the sweating sickness at the close of *A Book Against the Sweating Sickness* (1552) (in *The Thought and Culture of the English Renaissance: An Anthology of Tudor Prose, 1481–1555*, edited by Elizabeth M. Nugent, 301–02). John Taylor records its speed in 1625: "A healthful April, a diseased June / And dangerous July, brings all out of tune," 8. The following historians attest to the plague as uniquely horrific, a fact born out in early modern accounts: Shrewsbury, 5; Slack, *Impact of Plague*, 78; William J. Dohar, *The Black Death and Pastoral Leadership: The Diocese of Hereford in the Fourteenth Century*, 1; Paul Slack, Introduction to *Epidemics and Ideas: Essays on the Historical Perception of Pestilence*, eds. Terence Ranger and Paul Slack, 9; David Steel, 87. Lucinda McCray Beier discusses the direct impact plague had on legislation and upon continental medicine (*Sufferers and Healers: The Experience of Illness in Seventeenth-Century England*, 252). In his thorough and witty *History of the Royal College of Physicians of London*, Sir George Clark discusses plague as a factor in the founding of medical communities in England (2 vols. 1:54–60); Neil Samman shows by the example of Henry VIII some of the political repercus-sions of plague in "The Progresses of Henry the Eighth: 1509–1529," in *The Reign of Henry VIII: Politics, Policy and Piety*, edited by Diarmaid MacCullough, 69. See also Charles F. Mullett, *The Bubonic Plague and England*, 3. Alan Kreider in *English Chantries: the Road to Dissolution* (54–55) assesses the impact of plague upon the building of chantries.

8. Thomas Dekker, *The Wonderfull Yeare,* in *The Plague Pamphlets of Thomas Dekker,* edited by F. P. Wilson, 31–32. All citations of this poem will refer to pages from this edition.

9. See Slack's maps that mark London parishes visited by plague (*Impact of Plague,* 154–56). Savonarola and others asked, "Why does it commonly happen that in a town in which inhabitants are dying of plague, some of the people who are locked up, like monks or prisoners, remain untouched?" (quoted in Danielle Jacquart's "Theory, Everyday Practice and Three Fifteenth-Century Physicians," in *Renaissance Medical Learning: Evolution of a Tradition,* eds. Michael McVaugh and Nancy Siraisi, 145–46). William Rixton, a Londoner writing in 1592, expresses relief in a letter to his friend Crich in the country that the plague is "no nearer than the alleys as yet" (Herbert Berry, "A London Plague Bill for 1592, Crick and Goodwyffe Hurde," *English Literary Renaissance* 25.1 [Winter 1995]: 17–18).

10. William Bullein, *A dialogue bothe pleasaunte and pietifull wherein is a goodly regimente against the feuer pestilence with a consolacion and comfort against death / newly corrected by Willyam Belleyn, the autour thereof* (1564), 52. From this point on, all citations of this text will refer to pages from this edition. See the Introduction of this study, note 13, for an explanation of editions. Bullein had already shown his knowledge of the plague in a medical treatise, *A newe booke entituled the gouernement of healthe wherein is vttered manye notable rules for mannes preseruacion, with sondry symples and other matters, no lesse fruiteful then profitable: colect out of many approued authours. Reduced into the forme of a dialogue, for the better vnderstanding of thunlearned. Wherunto is added a sufferain regiment against the pestilence. By VVilliam Bulleyn* (1558).

11. Shrewsbury (37–39) and Dohar (1) note the devastation. See Nancy G. Siraisi's conclusion that "In fourteenth century Europe, plague was effectively a 'new' disease characterized by highly distinctive symptoms (at any rate in its bubonic form) and overwhelming, catastrophic impact. The experience of plague was sufficiently novel and terrifying to generate a new variety of medical literature, the plague tractate; 281 of these tractates giving explanations for the causes of plague and recommending treatment or precautions are known to have been composed between the mid-fourteenth century and 1500" (*Medieval and Early Renaissance Medicine,* 128). An interesting aside: Karlen posits that this pandemic halted the colonization of America by Norsemen, fundamentally changing the development of the Americas (*Man and Microbes,* 91). See also A. Lynn Martin, *Plague: Jesuit Accounts of Epidemic Disease in the Sixteenth Century,* 7.

12. The calculation of recovery is based on the mortality figures: 60–80 percent die from bubonic plague. Slack discusses recovery and

prolonged illness (176–77). Pollitzer estimates that one-half to two-thirds of Great Britain's population was lost to plague in the 1348–1349 visitation (15).

13. Horrox, Rosemary, ed., *Black Death*, 1994. Simultaneously a vivid testament to plague as it emerged in art, scholars conclude that "pestilence, like death, war and famine, is a universal theme" but that "the study of plague iconography is unique because it has a distinct beginning, the year 1347," and "bubonic plague is the only major illness for which an intricate iconography was developed" (Christine M. Boeckl, *Images of Plague and Pestilence: Iconography and Iconology*, 1).

14. Slack, 144. Slack adds that although fewer deaths resulted and a smaller geographical range was affected by the 1665–1666 plague, this one lasted longer, increasing the experienced level of suffering (176). On the other hand, there are those, like Steel, who entirely skip the plagues between the "Black Death" and "the Great Plague of London" (91).

15. Shrewsbury discusses in detail the Stratford-upon-Avon plague of 1563–1564, noting that from August to December of 1564, at least 175 citizens of the small town died. Shakespeare was born in April of that year, just prior to the greatest onslaught. See especially Shrewsbury's figure 30, which provides a graph of plague years in Stratford-upon-Avon (197).

16. Slack, 111, emphasis mine. See figure 3.

17. For a discussion of Langland, Chaucer, and bubonic plague, see Shrewsbury, 41–42. On Chaucer, see also Beidler's "The Plague and Chaucer's Pardoner," 257–92. On Boccaccio's and Petrarch's written response to plague, see Will Durant's *The Renaissance: A History of Civilization in Italy from 1304–1576 AD*, 21–22, 28–34, and see Steven M. Taylor, "Portraits of Pestilence: The Plague in the Works of Machaunt and Boccaccio," 105–18. On Erasmus, refer to Charles Creighton, 1:288–89. On Zwingli and the plague of 1519 and Luther in the 1527 plague, see Carter Lindberg, *European Reformations*, 177. For brief note on Holbein and Fletcher, see F. P. Wilson, *Plague in Shakespeare's London*, 172. On the Renaissance artist's range of plague-images available for refashioning, see Louise Marshall, "Manipulating the Sacred: Image and Plague in Renaissance Italy," 485–531. See also the very teachable book by Christine M. Boeckl.

Notes to Chapter Two

1. The majority of scholarly articles and books on early modern utopian projects attend to political contexts and purposes. See

Marina Leslie, *Renaissance Utopias and the Problem of History*, and Robert Appelbaum, *Literature and Utopian Politics*, for the most recent and useful of such accounts.

2. On the death rate of clergy, see Mullett, 20; Shrewsbury, 51–55; Slack, 193, 286; and Daniel Defoe, 183.

3. Bishop John Hooper, "Homily to be read in the time of Pestilence, 1563," in *Later Writings of Bishop Hooper*, edited by Charles Nevinson, Parker Society Publications 52, 167.

4. *A Looking-glasse for city and countrey vvherein is to be seene many fearfull examples in the time of this grieuous visitation, with an admonition to our Londoners flying from the city, and a perswasion [to the?] country to be more pitifull to such as come for succor amongst them* (1630); T. B., *A dialogue betuuixt a cittizen, and a poore countrey man and his wife, in the countrey, where the citizen remaineth now in this time of sicknesse written by him in the countrey, who sent the coppy to a friend in London; being both pitifull and pleasant* (1636); *Londons lamentation, or, A fit admonishment for city and countrey wherein is described certaine causes of this affliction and visitation of the plague, yeare 1641* (1641).

5. This injunction is still in existence: see Church of England, "The Communion of the Sick" in *The Annotated Book of Common Prayer*, edited by John Henry Blunt (London: Longmans, Green and Co., 1892), 472–74. For a lengthier discussion of flight and of those like Martin Luther and John Calvin who wrote to condemn it, see Slack, 41–44.

6. Henoch Clapham, *An epistle discoursing vpon the present pestilence Teaching what it is, and how the people of God should carrie themselues towards God and their neighbour therein. Reprinted with some additions. By Henoch Clapham* (1603), A3.

7. Privy Council, *Orders, thought meete by his Maiestie, and his Priuie Counsell, to be executed throughout the counties of this realme, in such townes, villages, and other places, as are, or may be hereafter infected with the plague, for the stay of further increase of the same by England and Wales* (1603). These orders are all but identical to those issued first in 1578 by Elizabeth I.

8. Quoted in Henoch Clapham, *Doctor Andros His Prosopopeia Answered* (1605), 8. All future references to this treatise are noted in the text by page number. Compare with Lancelot Andrewes, *A Sermon of the Pestilence Preached at Chiswick, 1603* (1636) in which Andrewes sounds more like Clapham, emphasizing the spiritual to the near neglect of the natural. This sermon was later printed in 1636. See chapter 9 for further discussion.

9. See the literary parallel to the Clapham-Andrewes debate in Thomas Dekker's *A rod for run-awayes Gods tokens, of his fearful iudgements, sundry wayes pronounced vpon this city, and on seuerall*

persons, both flying from it, and staying in it. Expressed in many dreadfull examples of sudden death . . . By Tho. D. (1625), and the response by B.V.: *The run-awyaes* [sic] *answer to a booke called, A rodde for runne-awayes. In vvhich are set downe a defense for their running, with some reasons perswading some of them neuer to come backe. The vsage of Londoners by the countrey people; drawne in a picture, artificially looking two waies, (foorth-right, and a-squint:) with an other picture done in lant-skipp, in which the Londoners and countrey-men dance a morris together. Lastly, a runne-awaies speech to his fellow run-awaies, arming them to meete death within the listes, and not to shunne him* (1625).

10. Thomas Lodge, *A treatise of the plague containing the nature, signes, and accidents of the same, with the certaine and absolute cure of the feuers, botches and carbuncles that raigne in these times: and aboue all things most singular experiments and preseruatiues in the same, gathered by the obseruation of diuers worthy trauailers, and selected out of the writing of the best learned phisitians in this age. By Thomas Lodge, Doctor in Phisicke* (1603), B3. All references to *A treatise of the plague* will refer to page numbers from this edition. The biblical verses included in Lodge's text are as follows, here taken from the King James Version: "Ye shall make you no idols nor graven image, neither rear you up a standing image, neither shall ye set up any image of stone in your land, to bow down unto it . . . If ye walk contrary unto me . . . I will bring seven times more plagues upon you according to your sins" (Leviticus 26.1–21); "But it shall come to pass, if thou wilt not hearken unto the voice of the Lord thy God, to observe to do all his commandments and his statutes which I command this day . . . the Lord shall make the pestilence cleave unto thee, until he have consumed thee from off the land, whither thou goest to possess it" (Deuteronomy 28.15–21).

11. Historians have until recently ignored the dynamic and sensible character of medieval and Renaissance medicine, focusing instead on surgery and on anatomy as the two "legitimate" forms of medicine practiced in early modern Europe. See Michael McVaugh and Nancy Siraisi, in the introduction to *Renaissance Medical Learning: Evolution of a Tradition*, 9. Another problem stems from the fashionable Foucauldian lens that views Galenic medicine and quarantine as one of many efforts to control the body and populations. For a response, see Michael C. Schoenfeldt, *Bodies and Selves in Early Modern England*.

12. Hippocrates never wrote of plague, *per se*, and while Galen's treatise on plague was lost and therefore unknown, "Nevertheless," V. Nutton states, "it was perfectly clear that Galen had known of the role of contagion, and of the part played in spreading disease by air that had become infected by the seeds of plague" ("Humanist

Surgery," *The Medical Renaissance of the Sixteenth Century*, edited by. A. Wear, R. K. French, and I. M. Lonine, 221).

13. For a discussion of contending medical theories on plague, see Walter Pagel, *Paracelsus: An Introduction to Philosophical Medicine in the Era of the Renaissance*, 172–89, and Wade Oliver, *Stalkers of Pestilence: The Story of Man's Ideas of Infection*, 49–123. Written in 1930, Wade's book is quite learned, covering theories on contagion with emphasis on plague from Hippocrates to Ehrlich in the nineteenth century, but its sound presentation is unfortunately disguised by the title.

14. For more on the power of mirth in plague-time, see Glending Olson, *Literature as Recreation in the Later Middle Ages*. Published just before study of the body and culture were in vogue, this important study has not received the attention it deserves.

15. See Rebecca Totaro, "Plague's Messengers: Communicating Hope and Despair in England 1500–1700," *The Journal of the Washington Academy of Science* 89: 1–2 (2003).

16. This work does not take Paracelsus into account, although Paracelsian medicine was a viable option by 1585. This may be due to what Slack and E. Cuvelier claim, that Lodge's treatise was actually a translation of a French treatise published 40 years earlier (see Slack, *Impact of Plague*, 24, and E. Cuvelier, "*A Treatise of the Plague de Thomas Lodge 1603*," *Etudes Anglaises* XXI (1968): 395–403). Knowledge of the treatise's origin, combined with the fact that we have evidence of its being published only one time, points to the relative insignificance of Lodge's treatise in terms of the marking of English concerns in 1603. Surprising numbers of scholars of English literature, however, rely on Lodge as the most essential source in their treatment of early modern English plague. This is likely due to Lodge's popularity from the prose work *Rosalynde*, now considered a source for Shakespeare's *As You Like It*. Nevertheless, Lodge was a practicing physician who remained in London during the plague and who would have known enough to add to the translated treatise as necessary.

17. Thomas Nashe, *Christs teares ouer Ierusalem Wherunto is annexed, a comparatiue admonition to London* (1593). For a more extensive account of the London plague house history, see F. P. Wilson, 74–84, to whom I am clearly indebted.

18. Sir Thomas Elyot, *The castel of helthe gathered, and made by Syr Thomas Elyot knight, out of the chief authors of phisyke; whereby euery man may knowe the state of his owne body, the preseruation of helthe, and how to instruct well his phisition in sicknes, that he be not deceyued* (1539), 88–89. On herbalists, see R. Palmer, "Pharmacy in the Republic of Venice in the Sixteenth Century," in *Medical Renaissance of the Sixteenth Century*, 105. See also Keith Thomas, *Religion and the Decline of Magic*, 11. Regimen

books were simplified forms of information contained primarily in the *Aphorisms and Prognostics of Hippocrates, Galen's Tegni* (also known as his *ars medica*), and the *Isagogue* of "Johannitus."

19. Pagel, *From Paracelsus to Van Helmont: Studies in Renaissance Medicine and Science,* edited by Marianne Winder, 454. See also Pagel's discussion of Paracelsus's and Van Helmont's views on humoral medicine in *The Religious and Philosophical Aspects of van Helmont's Science and Medicine,* Supplements to the Bulletin of the History of Medicine 2, 3–8.

20. For primary works, see George Chapman's *Bussy D'Ambois,* especially 3.2.442–48 and Shakespeare's *All's Well That Ends Well.* For scholarly examination of Paracelsianism in early modern English literature, there are only few treatments, and these include Henry D. Janowitz, "Helena's Medicine in *All's Well That Ends Well*: Is It Paracelsian or Hermetical in Origin?", *Cauda Pavonis: Studies in Hermeticism,* 20.1 (2001): 20–22; James R. Keller, "Paracelsian Medicine in Donne's 'Hymn to God, My God, in My Sickness'," *Seventeenth-Century News,* 59:1–2 (2001): 154–58; and Thomas Willard, "Donne's Anatomy Lesson: Vesalian or Paracelsian?" *John Donne Journal: Studies in the Age of Donne* 3:1 (1984): 35–61. If the amount of scholarship on Paracelsian theory in early modern English literature is any indication, it would seem that we must wait until the Romantics and Browning to have authors clearly championing Paracelsus. See Allen G. Debus, *The English Paracelsians.*

21. William Clowes, "The Epistle to the Reader," in *A right frutefull and approoued treatise, for the artificiall cure of that malady called in Latin Struma, and in English, the evill, cured by kinges and queenes of England Very necessary for all young practizers of chyrurgery. Written by William Clowes, one of her Maiesties chyrurgions, in the yeare of our Lord* (1602).

22. Even before Henry VIII had ascended to the throne, plague seemed to be tampering with his future power and even his lineage. In 1501 when Henry VII was king and Prince Henry's brother Arthur was betrothed to Catherine of Aragon, the plague nearly visited her before Arthur, or, later, Henry could. In a letter to the steward of her docking ship, King Henry VII writes, "the King's Grace, tenderly considering her great and long pain and travel upon the sea, would full gladly that she landed and lodged for the night at Gravesend; but forasmuch as the plague was there of late, and that is not yet clean purged thereof, the King would not that she should be put in any such adventure or danger, and therefore his Grace hath commanded the bark to be prepared and arrayed for her lodging" (quoted from the Harwick Papers in Creighton, 288; Creighton's research has proven invaluable for this part of my own). Remaining safely on board, Catherine avoided the plague at Gravesend that year, married Arthur,

and came to know and later marry that prince who would become Henry VIII. The Gravesend plague of 1501 was neither the first nor the last that would challenge Henry's reign and relationships.

23. Creighton, 288.

24. Neville Williams, *Henry the Eighth and his Court*, 108. Williams notes that the plague kept Anne and Henry apart in 1528, a fact appearing in their letters and one that may have contributed to their slight rate of conception (108). For companionship, Williams notes, Henry often kept the Venetian Friar Dennis Memmo shut up with him in Windsor (39).

25. Creighton, 293.

26. Shrewsbury, 162; Creighton, 301; see also Williams, 149.

27. Creighton (301) and Williams (162) attest to this absence of Henry at Edward's birth.

28. W. K. Jordan, *Edward the Sixth: The Young King*, 37.

29. Henry VIII, "Limiting the Attendance at Baptism of Prince Edward," in *Tudor Royal Proclamations: Volume One, The Early Tudors (1485–1553)*, edited by Paul L. Hughes and James F. Larkin, 259–60. This source includes many other proclamations related to plague. See proclamations numbered here, as in Hughes and Larkin, and with the year of their issue in the parentheses: 160 (1536), 223 (1543), 237 (1544), 293 (1547), 312 (1548). It is clear from the increase in the number of proclamations over time that Henry came more and more to use them as a defensive strategy. Still, he never established nationwide plague orders.

30. Francie Aidan Gasquet and Edmund Bishop, *Edward VI and the Book of Common Prayer*, 134; Creighton, 304.

31. For these and other proclamations, see Creighton but also the following: *By the Queene. A proclamation against bringing in of wines or other merchandise from Bourdeaux, in respect of the plague being there* (1585); *By the Queene. The Queenes most excellent Maiestie in her princely nature, considering how dangerous a matter it is by continuance of the faire called Bartholomew faire* (1593); *By the Queen's Commandment. For as much as it is found by good proof that many persons which have served of late on the seas in the journey towards Spain and Portugal, in coming from Plymouth and other ports of the realm have fallen sick by the way and diverse died as infected with the plague* (1589).

32. Elizabeth I, *Orders thought meete by her Majestie, and her privie Councell, to be executed throughout the Counties of this Realme, in such Townes, Villages, and other places, as are, or may be hereafter infected with the plague, for the stay of further increase of the same. Also, an advise set downe upon her Majesties expresse commaundement, by the best learned in Physicke within this Realme, contayning sundry good rules and easie medicines, without*

*charge to the meaner sort of people, as well for the preservation
of her good Subjects from the plague before infection, as for the
curing and ordring of them after they shalbe infected,* 1578.

33. See J. E. Neale's *Queen Elizabeth* for further record of some of
Elizabeth's encounters with plague. See also Edmund Grindal's
sermons delivered during the time (*The Remains of Edmund Grindal,
Successively Bishop of London and Archbishop of York and
Canterbury,* edited by William Nicholson, Parker Society Pub-
lications, 19).

34. See the following proclamations made by King James: *By the
King Forasmuch as it hath pleased God of his exceeding goodnesse,
to stay his heauy hand wherewith the last yeere hee punished our
city of London by the infection of the plague* (1604); and see *Orders,
thought meet by His Maiestie, and his Priuy Councell, to bee executed throughout the counties of this realm, in such townes,
uillages, and other places, as are, or may bee heerafter, infected with
the plague, for the stay of further increase of the same also, An aduice
set downe by the best learned physicke within this realme, containing sundry good rules and easie medicines, without charge to
the meaner sort of people, as well for the preseruation of his good
subjects from the plague before infection, as for the curing and ordering of them after they shall be infected* (1625). The latter is a
nearly word-for-word copy from Elizabeth's proclamation of essentially the same name from 1578. See Charles II, *By the King, a proclamation for a generall fast throughout this realm of England.
Sovereign* (1665) and *At the court at Oxford, the sixt of October
1665, present the King's Most Excellent Majesty . . . His Majesty taking into His Royall consideration and princely care the preventing
(by Gods blessing) as much as may be, any growth of the infection,
so dreadfully spread in other places from this his city of Oxford*
(1665). See also Cromwell's order, *Thursday the thirteenth of
August, 1657. At the Council at VVhite-hall. His Highness the Lord
Protector and his Privy Council, taking notice of the hand of God,
which at this time is gone out against this nation, in the present
visitation by sickness that is much spread over the land* (1657).

Notes to Chapter Three

1. Erasmus, *The Correspondence of Erasmus: Letters 142 to 297,
1501 to 1514,* 2 vols., trans. R. A. B. Mynors and D. F. S. Thomason,
2:252. The first letter we have in which Erasmus writes of plague is
from 1502: "The plague, which drove me to Louvain, still keeps me
there; Fortune has had a glorious fling at my expense this year!"
(2:59). All following letters of Erasmus are from this edition and

volume. Shrewsbury records the disbandment of lectures at Cambridge in 1513 and confirms Erasmus's isolation (2:160–61).

2. Erasmus, *Oration in Praise of the Art of Medicine: Declamatio in laudem artis medicae,* trans. Brian McGregor, in *Collected Works of Erasmus,* 29:46.

3. Erasmus, *The Correspondence,* 2:119. In 1514 Erasmus again declares that London's plague is so bad he dare not visit the city: "The plague is kindling sparks everywhere and looks like [it is] becoming a roaring blaze any day now" (2:283). In July of 1501 and September of 1502, in letters to Augustin Vincent and Willem Hermans respectively, Erasmus also recorded the impact of plague upon his plans (2: 37, 59).

4. On More's role as undersheriff and as commissioner of the sewers, see J. H. Hexter, *More's Utopia: Biography of an Idea,* 160; Arthur S. MacNalty, "Sir Thomas More as Public Health Reformer," in *Essential Articles for the Study of Thomas More,* edited by R. S. Sylvester and G. P. Marc'hadour, 126; Paul Slack, *The Impact of Plague,* 201. Hexter notes, in an appendix entitled "More as undersheriff," "I have been able to find no satisfactory account of the duties of the undersheriff in the sixteenth century. . . . There can be no doubt, in view of More's own statement, that it was as undersheriff of London that he represented the City's interests in litigation before the Royal Courts. The mechanics of this representation is perhaps indicated in the P.R.O lists of proceedings in Chancery, Star Chamber, etc., where in many instances it is the sheriffs rather than the Lord Mayor and Aldermen who are party to the suit" (160). See John Stow's *Survey of London,* which mentions undersheriffs in a marginal note: "Portgraves, since called shiriffes, and judges of the Kings Court, & have therefore under shiriffes men learned in the law, to sit in their Courts" (2:149).

5. Ernest L. Sabine, "Butchering in Medieval London," *Speculum* 8:3 (1933): 335–53.

6. Hexter notes, "Though much of the work [of the commissioner] was reparian in character and directed towards preventing the encroachment of the sea, flooding of law grounds and maintaining of river banks, regulations were also made against trade effluents, deposit of rubbish in rivers, and pollution of rivers, streams and wells" (125). In many ways, we might say that More was also commissioner of the air. See chapter 9 for details.

7. For information on More's role in the 1518 visitation, see Sir George Clark, *A History of the Royal College of Physicians of London,* 1:57–58. Creighton also discusses the context within which the orders of 1518 were created (2:290–91). Those orders took more permanent form under Elizabeth I in 1578, and they would endure well into the eighteenth century. When the *plaga* in England was no

longer bubonic plague, but cholera, visiting in the early nineteenth century, similar orders were issued. Quarantine laws were only enforced for these diseases in England.

8. Davies, 233.

9. Quoted in R. W. Chambers, *Thomas More*, 81. Chambers states, "More never wavered in his devotion to Catherine of Aragon" (81).

10. Some historians conclude that in 1502, Catherine's husband Prince Arthur died of plague while she herself caught plague and recovered. Albert DuBoys, in *Catherine of Aragon and the Sources of the English Reformation* (1:56–57), discusses the impact of the plague upon Catherine's life, although he does not mention the Gravesend plague which delayed her initial arrival in England. Of course there is debate over the cause of Arthur's death and Catherine's illness: "Most authors say that the young prince's health was delicate and gave way under the severity of winter," writes DuBoys, but, he goes on to state, "this is contradicted by the Spanish chroniclers, who derived their information from Catharine [sic] herself. They say he was strong and robust but was carried off suddenly by the plague, which was then prevalent in part of England. This statement is indirectly confirmed by the *Herald's Journal*, which, after describing the magnificent funeral of the prince at Worcester, mentions that at the very time of the ceremony the principal inhabitants of the city had assembled in the cathedral to deliberate on the measures to be taken against the prevalent disease" (56–57). It makes sense that, given the propensity to mask any shortcomings of the monarchy such as the prince's generally sickly condition, the court would wish to report that only the very most powerful of illnesses could kill royalty. The sweating sickness, on the other hand, was reputed to be easier to cure; moreover, records give no proof of its existence in London at the time. However, MacNalty is among the many that say that in 1502 Arthur "probably succumbed" to the Sweat and Catherine caught it but recovered (128).

11. By this time More was also in his second year as a barrister, thus taking time from that job to contemplate his life's vocation: to join a monastery, or to marry and become a lawyer as his father wished. The years of More's residence with the Carthusians cannot be precisely determined, but the common assumption is from 1501 to 1503 or 1504. Within this time, More would have known of Catherine's brush with death.

12. For more on the foundation of the Charterhouse and on its particular plague-time birth, see William F. Taylor, *The Charterhouse of London: Monastery, Palace, and Thomas Sutton's Foundation*, 1–6; Daniel Knowles and R. Neville Hadcock, *Medieval and Religious Houses: England and Wales*, 133; and John Stow, *Survey of London*, 2:81–82.

13. The Latin original is quoted in Stow, 2:81–82. Creighton translates the inscription (found in Stow) in order to gather data on the number of plague deaths in that year. He comes to the conclusion that the figures on the monument are exaggerated because the monument was not erected until 1371, when recollection and records may have been difficult to attain (Creighton 127–28).

14. E. E. Reynolds cites 1504 as the earliest year in which historians and biographers can prove — by means of a letter between More and Colet — that More knew Linacre (*The Field is Won: The Life and Death of Saint Thomas More* [London: Burns and Oates Ltd., 1968], 30).

15. In *Thomas Linacre*, William Osler confirms that "at Pavia in 1467 there were thirty-five teachers in the Medical faculty and at Padua quite as many," and "it was not until the third year of Edward VI, 1550, that the Oxford Lectureships were established" (39).

16. In "Physicians in Thomas More's Circle: The Impact of the New Learning on Medicine" (*Thomas Morus Jahrbuch, 1989*, 158–64), Gerhard Helmstaedter discusses More's contribution to his many friends in the field of medicine. See also Helmstaedter, "Health Equilibrium of the Utopians on Well-Being and Hygiene," *Thomas Morus Jahrbuch, 1992*. In *The English Hospital, 1070–1570*, Nicholas Orme and Margaret Webster discuss the history of monarchs who supported hospital projects (141). Orme and Webster discuss the Savoy in relation to Italian models (150). Helmsteadter notes the following in support of England's trend in imitating Italy: "Already Henry VII had appointed an Italian scholar to a Latin secretaryship, a position Andrea Ammonio in 1513 received from Henry VIII, the most intimate correspondent of Erasmus and also guest in More's house" (158). For a map of the Savoy palace and hospital, see Orme and Webster, 149.

17. For these definitions, see introduction, note 17.

18. Thomas More, *The Utopia*, in *The Complete Works of Thomas More*, eds. Edward Surtz and J. H. Hexter, 4:139. All references to *The Utopia* are to this edition and are cited by volume and page number.

19. The Surtz and Hexter notes to this passage say nothing of Sabine's article or of the original marginal note linking filth to plague. They do, nevertheless, discuss the authorship of the marginal notes and assign them to Erasmus, adding that it is likely that Giles had a hand in them as well (see the introduction).

20. Stow makes mention of the slow building of conduits in London, beginning in 1285 and still under construction by his time in 1583 (1:17).

21. Galen, *A Translation of Galen's Hygiene (De Sanitate Tuenda)*, 20. All following citations from Galen correspond to page numbers from this edition.

22. See *Utopia*, 4:182, including the marginal note at 182 (*Medicina utilissima*), and 4:120.

23. Orme and Webster, 17–18. On the required infirmaries within convents and monasteries, see also Lord Amultee's "Monastic Infirmaries" (in *The Evolution of Hospitals in Britain*, ed. F. N. L. Poynter), in which he draws evidence for his assessment of monastic infirmaries from the extensive rolls of Westminster Abbey, 1297–1536. These rolls are some of the few documents related to medieval infirmaries that are available (11–12).

24. See Amultee, 13. See also Orme and Webster who include floorplans from a number of infirmaries, showing the consistency in plan after plan — especially with regard to the central placement of the altar (88–91). The fact that all Cistercian abbeys and hospitals were built and operated in like manner supports the notion that convents and monasteries maintained more efficient, although not medical, facilities for care of the ill than any other at the time. On the Cistercians and on the rise of medical facilities in England prior to Thomas More's time, see Charles Talbot, *Medicine in Medieval England*, 172. Orme and Webster comment on the originally communal nature of the infirmary where brothers of all ranks slept, ate, and prayed together without indication of rank in the church. This began to change by the thirteenth century, but only where the architectural plan could accommodate separate chambers for clergy, laity, women, lepers, etc. (90–91).

25. Amultee, 13.

26. John Lennard, *But I Digress: The Exploitation of Parentheses in English Printed Verse*, 2.

27. Lennard explains that he selected Erasmus's terms "lunula(e)" in order to dicuss parenthetical statements, discussing the important relationship between the advent of humanism and the printing press (1).

28. More's use of lunulae in *Utopia* is a creative departure from the standard uses of the lunulae, and it differs from his use of them in *The History of Richard III*.

29. Another indication of More's view of lunulae as an important part of the narrative is his retention of them in his translation of Pico's work. In almost every case, he retains the lunulae in his translation in a manner identical to Pico's original — an approach different from that employed by editors of More's *Complete Works*. See Surtz and Hexter, 1:281–381.

30. See the Surtz and Hexter calculation of Utopian history: "The period of 1760 years carries us from AD 1516 to 244 BC" (4:120).

31. Lyman Tower Sargent defines "eutopia or positive utopia [as] — a nonexistent society described in considerable detail and normally located in time and space that the author intended a contemporaneous reader to view as considerably better than the society

in which that reader lived" ("Three Faces," 9). For a provocative, contemporary application and extension of the utopian terms in question (utopia, dystopia, eutopia, critical utopia, and so on), see Tom Moylan, *Demand the Impossible: Science Fiction and the Utopian Imagination* and also *Scraps of the Untainted Sky: Science Fiction, Utopia, Dystopia.*

Notes to Chapter Four

1. On the subject of the plague visitation and the dating of *Timon*, see A. L. Rowse, *William Shakespeare: A Biography*, 416; F. P. Wilson, 119–20; Honan, 347–49; and Barroll, 207. Because there is no record of the play being staged, the range of dates for its composition remains large. Barroll suggests it may have been written even after 1613.

2. Bloch, 1:5. See also the introduction.

3. Sir Walter Ralegh, *The discouerie of the large, rich, and bevvtiful empire of Guiana with a relation of the great and golden citie of Manoa (which the spanyards call El Dorado) and the prouinces of Emeria, Arromaia, Amapaia, and other countries, with their riuers, adioyning. Performed in the yeare 1595. by Sir W. Ralegh Knight, captaine of her Maiesties Guard, Lo. Warden of the Sannerries [sic], and her Highnesse Lieutenant generall of the countie of Cornewall* (1596), 81. For an examination of Ralegh's "interest in Guiana" being "much to the fore in these years" after the 1595 voyage and on its influence upon Shakespeare, see Rowse, *William Shakespeare: A Biography*, 264, and Louis B. Wright's *Gold, Glory and the Gospel: The Adventurous Lives and Times of Renaissance Explorers*, 271, 278–79, 285.

4. George Chapman, "De Guiana, Carmen Epicum," in *The Poems of George Chapman*, ll. 18–29. All following references to "*De Guiana*" are drawn from the above edition and refer to line numbers.

5. Included within Faye Marie Getz's publication of a medieval remedy book is one of many accounts of the multiple uses of gold (*Healing and Society in Medieval England: A Middle English Translation of the Pharmaceutical Writings of Gilbertus Anglicus*). Michael R. McVaugh makes mention of gold-based remedies used upon the Spanish king in 1318 (*Medicine Before the Plague: Practitioners and Their Patients in the Crown of Aragon, 1285–1345*, 35, 165). In *Studies in Medieval Science: Alchemy, Astrology, Mathematics, and Medicine*, Pearl Kibre discusses the concerns that Albertus Magnus expressed over alchemists' claims for the elixir-quality of transmuted gold (190–93).

6. Thomas Russel, *Diacatholicon Aureum or A generall powder of Gold, purging all offensive humours in mans bodie* (1602). The pages for this text are noted by letter, as in the original.

7. *The apologie, or defence of a verity heretofore published concerning a medicine called aurum potabile that is, the pure substance of gold, prepared, and made potable and medicinable without corrosiues, helpfully giuen for the health of man in most diseases, but especially auaileable for the strenghning* [sic] *and comforting of the heart and vitall spirits the perfomers of health: as an vniversall medicine. Together with the plaine, and true reasons . . . confirming the vniversalitie thereof. And lastly, the manner and order of administration or vse of this medicine in sundrie infirmities. By Francis Anthonie of London, doctor in physicke* (1616).

8. In *Sir Walter Ralegh: The Man and His Roles*, Stephen Greenblatt, among many others, confirms the unique value of Ralegh's venture. Although *The Discoverie* recorded fantastic peoples, places, and potential wealth, Ralegh's dream was "that which every man was willing to believe" (164).

9. William Shakespeare, *The Merry Wives of Windsor* in *The Arden Shakespeare Complete Works*, ed. Richard Proudfoot, Ann Thompson and David Scott Kastan, 1.3.66–67. All following in-text citations of Shakespeare's plays will be noted by act, scene, and line from this edition unless otherwise specified. For extended discussion of Shakespeare's allusion to Ralegh's venture in *Merry Wives*, see both works by Rowse, *Shakespeare the Man* (182) and *William Shakespeare: A Biography* (264).

10. Among the many scholars citing Ralegh's *Discoverie* as a source for both *Othello* and *The Tempest*, see Stephen W. May (*Sir Walter Ralegh*, 126) and Rowse (*Shakespeare the Man*, 255).

11. Ben Jonson, George Chapman, and John Marston, *Eastward Ho*, ed. C. G. Petter, 3.3.23–28. All quotations from this play refer to act, scene, and line from this edition.

12. Herford and Simpson likewise see the interesting combination of alchemy and El Dorado: "Alchemy was less affected by the religious revolutions of the age than by its eager scientific curiosity, its ingenious experimental art, its utopian economics. The prospect of generating gold from baser metals, which gave alchemic practices their tenacious hold upon the mass of men, lost none of its attractions in an age of eager enterprise, among men easily lured to the desert by the mirage of an El Dorado" (2:90). See also Rebecca Totaro, "Plague and Promise: Golden Destinations and a 'Ship of Fools' during the English Renaissance," in *Reading the Sea: New Essays on Sea Literature*, edited by Kevin Alexander Boon (New York: Fort Schuyler Press, 1999), 175–84.

13. One is inclined to look beyond the use of the word "plague" in the history plays, for with the exception of that in *Richard III*, we find it uttered largely as part of the cursing out of some rogue. Most often Falstaff is the one doing the swearing. This might be the subject of a paper on plague and cursing in early modern drama — "a plague on both your houses" and Webster's Duchess of Malfi's famous "Plagues, that make lanes through largest families, / Consume them" (edited by Elizabeth M. Brennan, 4.1.101–02) being most prominent. Plague does, over time, attain a more subtle role after early appearances in a morality play such as William Wager's *Enough is as Good as a Feast*.

14. For an investigation of prominent terms and themes in *Timon*, see Rolf Soellner's *Timon of Athens: The Pessimistic Tragedy*, 99–105.

15. Coppelia Kahn, "Magic of Bounty: *Timon of Athens*, Jacobean Patronage, and Maternal Power," *Shakespeare Quarterly* 38:1 (1987): 57. Kahn focuses on themes of bounty and usury in addition to power, gender, and identity. See also Rolf Soellner (104–05) who views sexual nausea as the primary image of disease in the play. If we were to focus more particularly on the sexual nature of this medium for plague, as many others have done, we would miss the significance of this scene in relation to the catalog of plagues that Timon's gold will fund.

16. William Shakespeare, *Timon of Athens*, ed. H. J. Oliver, *The Arden Shakespeare: The Complete Works*. Second edition, 1.1.281–85.

17. Shakespeare used the word "confound" and its various forms more often in *Timon of Athens* than in any of his other plays. It belongs with "plague" and "gold" through its frequent association with those terms.

18. John Taylor, *The fearefull summer*, 8.

19. For a more thorough discussion of Dekker's depiction of the Stalking Tamberlaine, see chapter 1, and see Dekker (*Wonderfull Yeare*, 31–32).

20. According to H. J. Oliver's Arden Shakespeare introduction to *Timon of Athens*, the sources from which Shakespeare most likely drew were North's translations of Plutarch's "Life of Alcibiades" and "Life of Marcus Antonius," and Lucian's *Timon, or the Misanthrope* (xxxii–xxxvii).

21. In North's translation of "Life of Marcus Antonius," Timon's presence in Athens got "everie man listening to heare what he would say, because it was a wonder to see him in that place." True to form, Timon tells the Athenians that they should all utilize his fig tree for hanging themselves (6:73).

22. Lucian, *Timon, or the Misanthrope*, 2:363.

23. What follows is a small selection of the many lines in the play linking air, breath, and disease: see 4.2.12–15, 4.2.20, 4.3.1–6, 4.3.109–11, 4.3.141–42, and 4.3.203–14.

24. For an interesting treatment of revenge plays as plague plays, see Melissa Smith, "The House, Sir, has been Visited: The Playhouse as Plaguehouse in Early Modern Revenge Tragedy," *The Journal of the Washington Academy of Science* 89: 1–2 (2003).

25. In many ways, this examination confirms G. Wilson Knight's assertion that Timon's longing for a golden world of social harmony is grounded in a forward-looking humanitarianism rather than in a backward-looking wish for a return to what was, whether that be to a feudal system, a golden age, or the womb (G. Wilson Knight, *The Wheel of Fire: Interpretations of Shakespearean Tragedy*, 210, 212, 239.). In such case, Timon stands alongside Lear, Hamlet, and Othello in his ability to imagine some of the heights of the human condition. At the beginning of the play, Timon sees the very best of humanity just as, in the beginning of their plays, Othello sees only the best of love and of Desdemona, Lear believes in love and in family, and Hamlet can see the divine in the dust. Timon might even be said to surpass some of these other tragic heroes in that he extended love of family beyond wife, mother, and daughter to include friendship with men and humanity in general. It is primarily family and even more specifically the female members of those families that bring down the other tragic heroes. Timon experiences betrayal at the hands of humanity at large, a humanity in which he is a part. This is the stuff of tragedy, the most ultimate and final kind. It seems clear, then, that those who dismiss Timon as either naive or as a scarcely drawn character miss *Timon*'s final tragic lesson. This tragedy is about far more than what critics, such as James C. Bulman claim: Timon's "naive assumption that an ideal community is possible at all" is the "deeper flaw in his character" (*The Heroic Idiom of Shakespearean Tragedy*, 135).

Notes to Chapter Five

1. Rosalind Miles, *Ben Jonson: His Life and Work*, 80; C. H. Herford, Percy Simpson, and Evelyn Simpson, eds., *Ben Jonson* (11 vols.), 1:52.

2. W. David Kay, *Ben Jonson: A Literary Life*, 2.

3. For mortality rates in the 1608–1609 visitation, see Wilson (118, 125), Slack (*Impact*, figure 6.1), and Creighton (1.494).

4. Ben Jonson, *The Alchemist*, edited by Elizabeth Cook, 1.1.110.

5. For an extensive assessment of Mammon and Subtle as messianic figures, see Robert M. Schuler's analysis of the similarities

between alchemy and Puritanism in "Jonson's Alchemists, Epicures, and Puritans," *Medieval & Renaissance Drama in England* 2, (1985): 171–208.

6. In defending Subtle, Mammon confirms the connection between the alchemist and his Paracelsian origins: "An excellent Paracelsian! And has done / Strange cures with mineral physic. He deals all / With spirits, he. He will not hear a word / Of Galen, or his tedious recipes" (2.3.230–33).

7. See act 1, scene 1 of Christopher Marlowe's *The Tragical History of Doctor Faustus* (in *Christopher Marlowe: Five Plays*, edited by Havelock Ellis, 133–96). In *Ben Jonson's Plays: An Introduction*, Robert E. Knoll discusses the difference between Marlowe's "hero" and Jonson's. He concludes, as I do in my comparison of Timon and Mammon, that Jonson does not see as tragic the Faustian and Timonian faith in overleaping the human (limited and fallen) condition (132). Later in the play, Surly sees Subtle as either a fraud or "the Faustus / That casteth figures, and can conjure, cures / Plague, piles, and pox, by the ephemerides, / And hold intelligence with all the bawds / And midwives of three shire" (4.6.35–49). I agree with Surley and scholars who consider Subtle to resemble Faustus; however, in comparing the conclusion of each drama and the apparent purposes of the authors, this resemblance falters.

8. See 5.5.77–80. Claude J. Summers and Ted-Larry Pebworth discuss the implications of Sir Epicure Mammon's knighthood in relation to the lower status of the other characters: the failure of his "Faustian vision" hurts the commonwealth in ways that the hopes of Dapper, Drugger, and the others never will (*Ben Jonson*, 87–88).

9. Mathew Martin, "Play and Plague in Ben Jonson's *The Alchemist*," *English Studies in Canada* 26.4 (2000): 397, 401.

10. Alan C. Dessen, *Jonson's Moral Comedy*, 132.

11. Ben Jonson, "XXXIII. To the Same," in *The Complete Poetry of Ben Jonson*, edited by William B. Hunter, Jr., 15. "ILe" is the correct spelling. See also William Drummond, *Notes of Conversations with Ben Jonson made by William Drummond of Hawthornden, January 1619*, in *Elizabethan and Jacobean Quartos*, ed. G. B. Harrison, 12.

12. "There is nothynge more ennemye to lyfe, than sorowe, callyd also heavynes, for it exhausteth the body" (64s), Thomas Elyot declared in *The castel of helthe* (1531); but by the same token, "Joye or gladnesse of harte dothe prolong the lyfe, it fatteth the body that is leane with troubles" (68t). For a more extensive discussion of mirth as a prescription for health in plague time, see chapter 2 — especially the sections treating William Bullein's Medicus (*A dialogue bothe pleasaunte and pietifull wherein is a goodly regimente against the feuer pestilence* [1564], 62) and Thomas Elyot's *The castel of helthe*. See also Glending Olson, *Literature as Recreation in the Later Middle*

Ages. From the *Regimen Sanitatis Salernis: or, The schoole of Salernes regiment of health*, a popular Renaissance training manual comes this refrain: "When Phisicke need, let these thy Doctors bee, Good dyet, quiet thoughts, heart mirthfull, free" (translated into English by Joannes de Mediolano in 1634 [3]). For further discussion of this influential regimen, see Mark D. Jordan, "The Construction of a Philosophical Medicine: Exegesis and Argument in Salernitian Teaching on the Soul," 42–61 in *Renaissance Medieval Learning*, ed. McVaugh and Siraisi.

Notes to Chapter Six

1. Paul Slack reports these years as having raised the mortality rates to extreme proportions (65), and in the introduction to the *Cambridge Companion to Bacon*, editor Markku Peltonen notes that plague kept Bacon from his studies at Cambridge during the months between August and March of 1574 (3).

2. Francis Bacon, Letter to Roger Palmer, in *The Works of Francis Bacon*, ed. James Spedding, Robert L. Ellis, and Douglas D. Heath, 14 vols, 14:534. All citations of Bacon will refer to volume and page number from this source. Slack records specific plague statistics for London during the years of Bacon's death (60). In 1625, 20 percent of London's population equalled roughly 26,000.

3. John Taylor, 8.

4. The following politicize the subject of early modern plague, often neglecting medical and historical approaches: see Eric Scott Mallin, *Inscribing the Time: Shakespeare and the End of the Elizabethan Era*; Cheryl Ross, "The Plague of the Alchemist" *Renaissance Quarterly* 41:3 (1988): 439–57; Sharon Achinstein, "Plagues and Publication: Ballads and the Representation of Disease in the English Renaissance," *Criticism* 34:1 (1992): 27–49.

5. Please see chapter 1 of this text, and compare with the certain signs listed by Davies, Pare, and Bullein.

6. Lisa Jardine, *Francis Bacon: Discovery and the Art of Discourse*, 137. Jardine further clarifies Bacon's understanding of similitude: "Physical similarity in objects may indicate a restricted similarity between further properties, and possibly similar origins and development. Resemblances between processes in different fields of investigation may indicate that both areas can be considered to be governed by the same collection of general rules, and thus that rules or principles commonly accepted as holding in one field may safely be assumed to hold in the other. The great advantage of such comparative techniques is that they are simple and immediate" (200–01).

7. For more on comic *A dialogue betuuixt a cittizen, and a poore countrey man and his wife,* see chapter 2 and figure 4.

8. Ben Jonson, *Volpone* in *Elizabethan Plays,* ed. Hazelton Spencer, 299–352.

9. Johnston, Arthur. *Francis Bacon,* 159–60.

10. *De Augmentis,* in *The Works of Francis Bacon,* 5:437.

11. James Stephens, *Francis Bacon and the Style of Science,* 157.

12. Here follows the only commentary on this paper in Spedding, Ellis, and Heath: "This paper follows the *New Atlantis* in the original edition, and concludes the volume" (3:167). I have been unable to find any mention of it elsewhere, but in brief, attached as an afterthought to discussions of the *New Atlantis*; for example, see Peter Zagorin, *Francis Bacon,* 46. Zargorin mentions but does not comment upon the context of the *Magnalia,* and he does not record it among Bacon's works in the index.

Notes to Chapter Seven

1. Katie Whitaker, *Mad Madge: The Extraordinary life of Margaret Cavendish, Duchess of Newcastle, the First Woman to Live by her Pen,* xiii.

2. Margaret Cavendish, "A World in an Eare-Ring," *Poems and Fancies* (1653), lix.

3. *Philosophical and Physical Fancies* (1653). All citations of this text will refer to pages from this edition.

4. *The World's Olio* (1655), 162. All citations of this text will refer to pages from this edition. According to Whitaker, she published the work close to the end of 1654 (180).

5. *Philosophical and Physical Opinions* (1655), 143. All citations of this text will refer to pages from this edition.

6. *Philosophical and Physical Observations* (1663), 143. All citations of this text will refer to pages from this edition.

7. The term "loimotia" is rare for the period, and there is no entry for it in the Oxford English Dictionary. Based on the entry for "loimography," it means essentially, the science of treating pestilential disease — a term that dates from the early eighteenth century and was used with slightly greater frequency in the mid nineteenth century.

8. See *CCXI sociable letters written by the thrice noble, illustrious, and excellent princess, the Lady Marchioness of Newcastle* (1663) and *Philosophical letters, or, Modest reflections upon some opinions in natural philosophy maintained by several famous and learned authors of this age, expressed by way of letters / by the thrice noble, illustrious, and excellent princess the Lady Marchioness of Newcastle* (1664).

9. For more on the Cavendish circle, including Margaret's relationships with Hobbes and Descartes, Whitaker is a reasonable point of entry into an ongoing scholarly inquiry.

10. Margaret Cavendish, *The Description of a New World, Called the Blazing World*, in *The Blazing World and Other Writings*, edited by Kate Lilley, 158. All subsequent references to *The Blazing World* are from this edition.

11. It is interesting that Cavendish makes the following groupings: the bear-men are the experimental philosophers whom she disbands when they rely too heavily on telescopes and microscopes (*The Blazing World*, 144–45); the ape-men are her chemists, who see the Paracelsian human elements of salt, sulfur, and mercury replacing Galen's humors (148). She makes the bird-men her astronomers and the satyrs her Galenic physicians, whom she belittles to a lesser degree than the rest (134, 154–55, 158).

Notes to Chapter Eight

1. *Observations upon experimental philosophy to which is added, The description of a new blazing world* (1666), C. Only two years later did Cavendish publish *The Blazing World* separately, and in her letter "To the Ladies" that introduces the reissued work, she explains, "This present Description of a New World; was made as an Appendix to my Observations upon Experimental Philosophy; and, having some Sympathy and Coherence with each other, were joyned together as Two several Worlds, at their Two Poles. But, by reason most Ladies take no delight in Philosophical Arguments, I separated some from the mentioned Observations, and caused them to go out by themselves, that I might express my Respects, in presenting to Them such Fancies as my Contemplations did afford" (In *The description of a new world, called the blazing-world / written by the thrice noble, illustrious, and excellent princesse, the Duchess of Newcastle* [1668].)

2. Schuler, *Francis Bacon and Scientific Poetry*, 9. Schuler speaks of "Lucretius, whose long poem was available to [Bacon] intact and whom he cites more often than the others" (42), showing that Lucretius was indeed a favorite of Bacon.

3. Lucretius, *De Rerum Natura*, trans. R. H. D. Rouse, 1:935–50.

4. Mary-Rose Sargent, "Bacon as an Advocate for Cooperative Scientific Research," in *The Cambridge Companion to Bacon*, edited by Markku Peltonen, 152.

5. See Denise Albanese's chapter, "*The New Atlantis*, and the Uses of Utopia," in her book *New Science, New World*, 92–120. Albanese develops her argument in order to explain the differences between Thomas More's *Utopia*, which, for example, allows for the

inclusion of a sexual inspection, and Bacon's *New Atlantis*, which entirely squelches the erotic (118–20).

6. See John Channing Briggs, "Bacon's Science and Religion," in *The Cambridge Companion to Bacon*, edited by Peltonen; and Briggs, *Francis Bacon and the Rhetoric of Nature*.

7. Anna Battigelli, *Margaret Cavendish and the Exiles of the Mind*, 102. In "Producing Petty Gods: Margaret Cavendish's Critique of Experimental Science," Eve Keller observes, "When it is considered in light of her *Observations*, the *Blazing World* is routinely treated as Cavendish's apologetic retreat: unable to make a believable mark in the 'real' and difficult world of fact, the argument goes, Cavendish escaped to the easy world of fiction. But to my mind, the *Blazing World* actually continues the critique of experimental science begun in the *Observations*" (*English Literary History* 64 [1997], 459).

8. Collette V. Michael, introduction to *The Grounds of Natural Philosophy* by Margaret Cavendish, xvi.

9. John Rogers, *The Matter of Revolution: Science, Poetry, and Politics in the Age of Milton*. Rogers discusses Cavendish's theories on matter only as they are finally related to gender and to Cavendish's program for raising the status of women; see especially 181, 185, 188, 201–03.

10. Battigelli, 114. In this regard, Battigelli might see Cavendish as more like Robert Burton, who also used science to justify a discussion of "mind"; however, I see Burton quite differently. He uses science to complement if not make somewhat less overt his more religious quest for the cure of melancholy — a condition he believed resulted from separation from God. Cavendish does not depict melancholy in her utopia, although she suffered from it; nor does she explore science in order to discuss faith.

11. William Rawley, "To the Reader," in *The Works of Francis Bacon*, ed. Spedding, Ellis, and Heath, 3:127.

12. Arthur Johnston, *Francis Bacon*, 147.

13. In *Francis Bacon and Scientific Poetry*, Robert Schuler discusses this seeming paradox and provides us with reason enough to conclude that Bacon would have rather strongly disliked Cavendish's version of natural philosophy: "[Bacon] adopted stylistic eloquence, poetic similitudes, and 'cultivated' language generally as 'instruments' for *presenting* his new scientific program (especially to a wide audience) — at the same time he insisted that 'the sons of science' should use wholly 'style-less' language for expression of 'objective scientific truth'" (55). "Fable" is after all quite distinct from "fancy," because it is an instrument used in the service of science.

14. John Channing Briggs, "Bacon's Science and Religion," 176–77.

15. On Cavendish's understanding of death, see *Observations Upon Experimental Philosophy,* 331, 333, 346, 352, 354.

16. By the time Cavendish was writing, Abraham Cowley had expressed an overwhelming appreciation of Bacon in "To the Royal Society": "From these and all long errors of the way / In which our wandering predecessors went, / And like th'old Hebrews, many years did stray / In deserts but of small extent / Bacon, like Moses, led us forth at last / The barren wilderness he past, / Did on the very border stand / Of the blest promis'd land, / And from the mountain's top of his exalted wit, / Saw it himself, and shew'd us it." Cavendish would have argued to the contrary that not only was Bacon no Moses, but also his program of science could no more "press into the privatest recess" of nature and transform "her" into a humbled handmaid spinning gold for mankind than Bacon could himself find the philosopher's stone or the cure for plague.

17. For a discussion of Cavendish's anger at those making what she thought to be arrogant claims regarding the nature of humans, see Katie Whitaker, 141, 288, and see each of Cavendish's treatises on natural philosophy but especially those written later in her career.

Notes to Chapter Nine

1. See Aristotle, *On Respiration, The Complete Works of Aristotle: The Revised Oxford Translation,* 748–49. See also Aristotle, *On Breath* in the same volume, 764–73.

2. Adequately regulated internal heat aided in digestion, as food taken in was transmuted by means of the heat into the appropriate humors. If the air one inhaled was pure, self-regulated, or regulated by some sort of technology, then one's life span would only increase. See William Kerrigan's well-known treatment of digestion in Milton's works: *The Sacred Complex: On the Psychogenesis of* Paradise Lost.

3. In More's *Utopia,* for example, Raphael describes Utopian infrastructure: "Outside the city are designated places where all gore and offal may be washed away in running water. From these places they transport the carcasses of animals slaughtered and cleaned by the hands of slaves" (4:139). Raphael explains in greater detail that the Utopians simply "do not permit to be brought inside the city anything filthy or unclean for fear that the air, tainted by putrefaction, should engender disease" (4:139). See also Bacon's *New Atlantis,* where the inhabitants have harnessed the winds, his treatment of plague in *The Natural History* (especially chapter 6), and Robert Burton's "Digression of Air" in *The Anatomy of Melancholy,* Floyd Dell and Paul Jordan-Smith, eds.

4. It is noteworthy that Robert Boyle began his exhaustive study of the air in this time, and it is worth reconsidering his lesser known work on pneumatics: *An Experimental Discourse of some Unheeded Causes of the Insalubrity and Salubrity of the Air, Being a Part of an Intended Natural History of Air* (1690). Boyle's first published account of pneumatics dates from 1660.

5. John Evelyn, *Fumifugium: or, The Inconveniencie of the Aer and Smoak of London Dissipated* (1661).

6. The problem of foul-smelling air in plague-time is well documented, dating to as early as 1391 if not earlier. Ernest L. Sabine's venerable study "Butchering in Medieval London" confirms that during plague-time, people grew even more concerned with the general dumping of waste in their waterways and streets. Many people simply emptied their waste upon the most convenient pile, but during plague visitations, Londoners grew less tolerant of butchers and the lack of sanitary practices. They complained directly to their officials and were taken seriously. As early as 1391 when plague again visited London, her inhabitants protested against the butchery practices, and in December of that year the king notified the mayor and the sheriffs of London that the city would be penalized if streets and waterways were not kept clean. By 1470 the complaints were still mounting in response to ditches and rivers blocked. As a remedy, Evelyn suggests that the king relocate certain industries outside of the city and plant gardens like a moat around it, so that the perfumed blossoms will counter the smoke.

7. The words themselves are worth considering: inhale, exhale, expire, inspire, and aspire — with the latter meaning to breathe after or to pant after, which is quite appropriate for Satan and the hell hounds.

8. John Milton, *Paradise Lost*, in *John Milton: The Complete Poems and Major Prose*, edited by Merritt Y. Hughes, 1.222–38. All future citations of *Paradise Lost* are from this edition and refer to book and line number.

9. See Rogers (148), who intentionally follows Kerrigan in his reading here.

10. Because of the change in the orientation of planets, "Beast now with Beast gan war, and Fowl with Fowl, / And fish with fish" (10.710–11).

11. See also *Paradise Lost* 9.193–99 for the general breath of life exhaled by all created things — an exhalation sent to the Creator whose "nostrils fill/ With grateful smell."

12. See Revelation, chapter 8 in particular. It is interesting to note that Andrewes's sermon was printed in 1636, ten years after Milton wrote an elegy on Andrewes. One wonders if Milton read this

sermon. He did not agree with Andrewes's conservative interpretation of the Bible and argued against Andrewes by name in several chapters of *The Reason of Church Government* (in Hughes, 640–89). Yet the date of *Reason of Church Government*, published in 1642, argues for Milton's knowledge of Andrewes's full body of work.

13. Elizabeth I, *Orders thought meete by her Majestie, and her privie Councell, to be executed throughout the Counties of this Realme, in such Townes, Villages, and other places, as are, or may be hereafter infected with the plague, for the stay of further increase of the same. Also, an advise set downe upon her Majesties expresse commaundement, by the best learned in Physicke within this Realme, contayning sundry good rules and easie medicines, without charge to the meaner sort of people, as well for the preservation of her good Subjects from the plague before infection, as for the curing and ordring of them after they shalbe infected,* 1578. See chapter 2 of this book.

14. See among others Nathaniel Henshaw, *Aero-chalinos, Or, the Regifter for the Air; in five Chapters.* Dublin, 1664. Henshaw recommends an air pump for the rectification of health brought about by altering the air in a room in the home and creating as it were an immediate change in climate.

15. Michael A Lev, "Chinese Turn to Herbs to Root Out SARS," in *The Chicago Tribune,* http://www.apria.com/resources/1,2725,494-26998,00.html, available April 11, 2003; http://www.yourvitalhealth.com/news/vfn102.cfm, available September 23, 2004.

16. Before we conclude that "China is different," we should look to the United States Food and Drug Administration website warning consumers in the United States to beware of SARS remedy scams including pill and air purifying products ("FTC and FDA Crackdown on Internet Marketers of Bogus SARS Prevention Products," in *FDA News* http://www.fda.gov/bbs/topics/NEWS/2003/NEW00904.html, available September 23, 2004).

Notes to Conclusion

1. Department of Health and Human Services, *Center for Disease Control and Prevention,* http://www.cdc.gov/, cited September 22, 2004; Health Canada, *Health Canada Online,* http://www.hc-sc.gc.ca/english/, cited September 22, 2004; Department of Health, *Welcome to the Department of Health,* http://www.dh.gov.uk/Home/fs/en, cited September 22, 2004; World Health Organization, http://www.who.int/en/, cited September 22, 2004. Here I note, too

late and too quickly for my comfort on some level, the fact that the "we" this book intends is the we who can afford the luxury of living beyond plague-time. Those living in countries or even pockets of countries ravaged by AIDS and prone to outbreaks of cholera, diptheria, and yellow fever are not "us" in this case. They are not beyond plague-time. Their hope for a healthier world, however, may indeed be greater. Their utopian plans may be more important and more legitimate.

2. Each of the following webpages were accessible as recently as September 22, 2004: the World Health Organization, "Plague," http://www.who.int/health_topics/plague/en/; Centers for Disease Control, "Health Topic: Plague," http://www.cdc.gov/health/plague.htm; Department of Health, "Plague," http://www.dh.gov.uk/PolicyAnd Guidance/HealthAndSocialCareTopics/Plague/fs/en; Health Canada, "Emergency Preparedness: The Plague," http://www.hc-sc.gc.ca/english/epr/plague.html.

3. Centers for Disease Control and Prevention, "National Center for Infection Disease. Travelers' Health: Plague," http://www.cdc.gov/travel/diseases/plague.htm. September 22, 2004.

Works Cited

Achinstein, Sharon. "Plagues and Publication: Ballads and the Representation of Disease in the English Renaissance." *Criticism* 34:1 (1992): 27–49.

Albanese, Denise. *New Science, New World.* Durham, N.C.: Duke University Press, 1996.

Amultee, Lord. "Monastic Infirmaries." In *The Evolution of Hospitals in Britain,* edited by F. N. L. Poynter, 1–26. London: Pitman Medical, 1964.

Andrewes, Lancelot. *A Sermon of the Pestilence Preached at Chiswick, 1603.* 1636.

Anthonie, Francis. *The apologie, or defence of a verity heretofore published concerning a medicine called aurum potabile that is, the pure substance of gold, prepared, and made potable and medicinable without corrosiues, helpfully giuen for the health of man in most diseases, but especially auaileable for the strenghning [sic] and comforting of the heart and vitall spirits the perfomers of health: as an vniversall medicine. Together with the plaine, and true reasons . . . confirming the vniversalitie thereof. And lastly, the manner and order of administration or vse of this medicine in sundrie infirmities. By Francis Anthonie of London, doctor in physicke.* 1616.

Appelbaum, Robert. *Literature and Utopian Politics in Seventeenth-Century England.* Cambridge: Cambridge University Press, 2002.

Aristotle. *On Breath.* In *The Complete Works of Aristotle: The Revised Oxford Translation,* edited by Jonathan Barnes, 764–73. Princeton: Princeton University Press, 1984.

———. *On Youth, Old Age, Life and Death, and Respiration*. In *The Complete Works of Aristotle: The Revised Oxford Translation*, 745–63.

B. V. *The run-awyaes answer to a booke called, A rodde for runne-awayes. In vvhich are set downe a defense for their running, with some reasons perswading some of them neuer to come backe. The vsage of Londoners by the countrey people; drawne in a picture, artificially looking two waies, (foorth-right, and a-squint:) with an other picture done in lant-skipp, in which the Londoners and countrey-men dance a morris together. Lastly, a runne-awaies speech to his fellow run-awaies, arming them to meete death within the listes, and not to shunne him*. 1625.

Bacon, Francis. *De Augmentis*. In *The Works of Francis Bacon*, 14 vols., edited by James Spedding, Robert L. Ellis, and Douglas D. Heath, 5:275–498. London: Longman, 1857–1874; rpt. New York: Garrett Press, 1968.

———. "Letter to Mr. Roger Palmer." In *The Works of Francis Bacon*, 14 vols., edited by James Spedding, Robert L. Ellis, and Douglas D. Heath, 14:534. London: Longman, 1857–1874; rpt. New York: Garrett Press, 1968.

———. "*Magnalia Naturae: Praecipue Quoad Usus Humanos*." In *The Works of Francis Bacon*, 14 vols., edited by James Spedding, Robert L. Ellis, and Douglas D. Heath, 3:167–68. London: Longman, 1857–1874; rpt. New York: Garrett Press, 1968.

———. *The New Atlantis*. In *The Works of Francis Bacon*, 14 vols., edited by James Spedding, Robert L. Ellis, and Douglas D. Heath, 3:129–66. London: Longman, 1857–1874; rpt. New York: Garrett Press, 1968.

———. *Sylva Sylvarum: or The Natural History in Ten Centuries*. In *The Works of Francis Bacon*, 14 vols., edited by James Spedding, Robert L. Ellis, and Douglas D. Heath, 2:339–672. London: Longman, 1857–1874; rpt. New York: Garrett Press, 1968.

Barroll, Leeds. *Politics, Plague, and Shakespeare's Theater: The Stuart Years*. Ithaca, N.Y.: Cornell University Press, 1991.

Battigelli, Anna. *Margaret Cavendish and the Exiles of the Mind*. Lexington: University Press of Kentucky, 1998.

Beidler, Peter G. "The Plague and Chaucer's *Pardoner*." *The Chaucer Review* 16:3 (1982): 257–92.

Beier, Lucinda McCray. *Sufferers and Healers: The Experience of Illness in Seventeenth-Century England.* London: Routledge and Kegan Paul, 1987.

Berry, Herbert. "A London Plague Bill for 1592, Crich and Goodwyffe Hurde." *English Literary Renaissance* 25:1 (1995): 3–25.

Bloch, Ernst. *The Principle of Hope.* 3 vols. Cambridge, Mass.: MIT Press, 1986.

Boeckl, Christine M. *Images of Plague and Pestilence: Iconography and Iconology.* Sixteenth Century Essays and Studies 53. Missouri: Truman State University Press, 2000.

Bower, Rick. "Antidote to the Plague: Thomas Dekker's Story-telling in *The Wonderful Year* (1603)." *English Studies* 73:3 (1992): 229–39.

Boyle, Robert. *An Experimental Discourse of some Unheeded Causes of the Insalubrity and Salubrity of the Air, Being a Part of an intended Natural History of Air.* 1690.

Brewer, Thomas. *A dialogue betuuixt a cittizen, and a poore countrey man and his wife, in the countrey, where the citizen remaineth now in this time of sicknesse written by him in the countrey, who sent the coppy to a friend in London; being both pitifull and pleasant.* 1636.

Briggs, John Channing. "Bacon's Science and Religion." In *The Cambridge Companion to Bacon,* edited by Markku Peltonen, 173–99. Cambridge: Cambridge University Press, 1996.

———. *Francis Bacon and the Rhetoric of Nature.* Cambridge: Cambridge University Press, 1989.

Bruce, John. "Milton's Mephitic Muse: Plague, Religion and the Infection Metaphor of *Paradise Lost*." *Journal of Evolutionary Psychology* 18:3–4 (1997): 238–48.

Bullein, William. *A dialogue bothe pleasaunte and pietifull wherein is a goodly regimente against the feuer pestilence with a consolacion and comfort against death / newly corrected by Willyam Belleyn, the autour thereof.* 1564.

———. *A Dialogue Against the Fever Pestilence .* 1578. Edited by Mark W. Bullen and A. H. Bullen. Early English Text Society 52. New York: Trubner, 1888.

———. *A newe booke entituled the gouernement of healthe wherein is vttered manye notable rules for mannes preseruacion, with sondry symples and other matters, no lesse fruiteful then profitable: colect out of many approued authours. Reduced into the forme of a dialogue, for the better vnderstanding of thunlearned. Wherunto is added a sufferain regiment against the pestilence. By VVilliam Bulleyn.* 1558.

Bulman, James C. *The Heroic Idiom of Shakespearean Tragedy.* Newark: University of Delaware Press, 1985.

Burton, Robert. *The Anatomy of Melancholy.* 1628. Edited by Floyd Dell and Paul Jordan-Smith. New York: Tudor, 1927.

Canada Health. "Emergency Preparedness: The Plague." In *Health Canada.* http://www.hc-sc.gc.ca/english/epr/plague.html. Accessed September 22, 2004.

Cantor, Norman. *In the Wake of Plague: Black Death and the World it Made.* New York: The Free Press, 2001.

Cauis, John. *A Book Against the Sweating Sickness.* 1552. In *The Thought and Culture of the English Renaissance: An Anthology of Tudor Prose, 1481–1555,* edited by Elizabeth M. Nugent, 301–02. Cambridge: Cambridge University Press, 1955.

Cavendish, Margaret. "A World in an Eare-Ring." 1653. In *Poems and Fancies,* lix. Providence: Brown University Women Writers Project, 1993.

———. *Philosophical and Physical Fancies.* 1653.

———. *The World's Olio.* 1655. Providence, R.I.: Brown University Women Writers Project, 1993.

———. *Philosophical and Physical Opinions.* 1655.

———. *CCXI sociable letters written by the thrice noble, illustrious, and excellent princess, the Lady Marchioness of Newcastle.* 1663.

———. *Philosophical and Physical Opinions.* 1663.

———. *Philosophical letters, or, Modest reflections upon some opinions in natural philosophy maintained by several famous and learned authors of this age, expressed by way of letters / by the thrice noble, illustrious, and excellent princess the Lady Marchioness of Newcastle.* 1664.

———. *Observations Upon Experimental Philosophy: To Which is added, the Description of a New Blazing World.* 1666.

———. *The Description of a New World Called the Blazing World.* 1666. In *The Blazing World and Other Writings,* edited by Kate Lilley, 125–202. London: Penguin Classics, 1994.

———. *The Grounds of Natural Philosophy.* 1668. Edited by Collette V. Michael. Women in the Sciences 2. West Cornwall, Conn.: Locust Hill Press, 1996.

———. "To the Ladies." In *The description of a new world, called the blazing-world written by the thrice noble, illustrious, and excellent princesse, the Duchess of Newcastle.* 1668.

Centers for Disease Control and Prevention. "Health Topic: Plague." http://www.cdc.gov/health/plague.htm. Accessed September 22, 2004.

———. "National Center for Infection Disease: Travelers' Health: Plague." http://www.cdc.gov/travel/diseases/plague.htm. Accessed September 22, 2004.

Chambers, R. W. *Thomas More.* Ann Arbor: University of Michigan Press, 1965.

Chapman, George. *Bussy D'Ambois.* Edited by Robert J. Lordi. Lincoln: University of Nebraska Press, 1962.

———. "*De Guiana, Carmen Epicum.*" In *The Poems of George Chapman*, edited by Phyllis Brooks Bartlett, 353–57. New York: Russell and Russell, 1962.

———. "The Communion of the Sick." In *The Annotated Book of Common Prayer*, edited by John Henry Blunt, 472–74. London: Longmans, Green, 1892.

Charles II, *At the court at Oxford, the sixt [sic] of October 1665, present the King's Most Excellent Majesty . . . His Majesty taking into His Royall consideration and princely care the preventing (by Gods blessing) as much as may be, any growth of the infection, so dreadfully spread in other places from this his city of Oxford.* 1665.

———. *By the King, a proclamation for a generall fast throughout this realm of England.* Sovereign. 1665.

Cipolla, Carlo M. *Fighting the Plague in Seventeenth-Century Italy.* The Curti Lectures. Madison: University of Wisconsin Press, 1981.

Claeys, Gregory and Lyman Tower Sargent, Editors. *The Utopia Reader.* New York: New York University Press, 1999.

Clapham, Henoch. *An epistle discoursing vpon the present pestilence Teaching what it is, and how the people of God should carrie themselues towards God and their neighbour therein. Reprinted with some additions. By Henoch Clapham.* 1603.

————. *Doctor Andros His Prosopopeia Answered.* 1605.

Clark, Sir George. *History of the Royal College of Physicians of London.* Vol. 1. Oxford: Clarendon Press, 1964.

Clowes, William. "The Epistle to the Reader." In *A right frutefull and approoued treatise, for the artificiall cure of that malady called in Latin Struma, and in English, the evill, cured by kinges and queenes of England Very necessary for all young practizers of chyrurgery.* 1602.

Cowley, Abraham, "To the Royal Society." In *The History of the Royal-Society of London,* by Thomas Spratt. 1667.

Creighton, Charles. *A History of Epidemics in Britain.* 2 vols. Cambridge: Cambridge University Press, 1891–1894.

Cromwell, Sir Oliver. *Thursday the thirteenth of August, 1657. At the Council at VVhite-hall. His Highness the Lord Protector and his Privy Council, taking notice of the hand of God, which at this time is gone out against this nation, in the present visitation by sickness that is much spread over the land.* 1657.

Cuvelier, E. "*A Treatise of the Plague de Thomas Lodge 1603.*" *Etudes Anglaises* 21 (1968): 395–403.

Davies, John. *Humours heau'n on earth with the ciuile warres of death and fortune. As also the triumph of death: or, the picture of the plague, according to the life; as it was in anno Domini 1603.* 1609.

Debus, Allen G. *The English Paracelsians.* London: Oldbourne Booke Co., 1965.

Defoe, Daniel. *A Journal of the Plague Year.* A Norton Critical Edition. Edited by Paula R. Backscheider. New York: W. W. Norton, 1992.

Dekker, Thomas. *The Wonderfull Yeare.* 1603. In *The Plague Pamphlets of Thomas Dekker,* edited by F. P. Wilson, 9–61. Oxford: Clarendon Press, 1925.

————. *A rod for run-awayes Gods tokens, of his feareful iudgements, sundry wayes pronounced vpon this city, and on seuerall persons, both flying from it, and staying in it. Expressed in many dreadfull examples of sudden death . . . By Tho. D.* 1625.

Department of Health, "Plague." http://www.dh.gov.uk/PolicyAnd Guidance/HealthAndSocialCareTopics/Plague/fs/en. Accessed September 22, 2004.

Dessen, Alan C. *Jonson's Moral Comedy*. Chicago: Northwestern University Press, 1971.

Dohar, William J. *The Black Death and Pastoral Leadership: The Diocese of Hereford in the Fourteenth Century*. Middle Ages Series. Philadelphia: University of Pennsylvania Press, 1995.

Drummond, William. *Notes of Conversations with Ben Jonson made by William Drummond of Hawthornden, January 1619*. Elizabethan and Jacobean Quartos. Edited by G. B. Harrison. New York: Barnes and Noble, 1966.

Du Boys, Albert. *Catherine of Aragon and the Sources of the Reformation*. 2 vols. in 1. New York: Burt Franklin, 1968.

Duncan-Jones, Katherine. *Ungentle Shakespeare: Scenes from his Life*. London: Arden Shakespeare, 2001.

Durant, Will. *The Renaissance: A History of Civilization in Italy from 1304–1576 AD*. New York: Simon and Schuster, 1953.

Edwards, Karen L. "The Balm of Life." In *Milton and the Natural World: Science and Poetry in* Paradise Lost, 182–98. Cambridge: Cambridge University Press, 1999.

Eliav-Feldon, Miriam. *Realistic Utopias: The Ideal Imaginary Societies of the Renaissance, 1516–1630*. Oxford Historical Monographs. Oxford: Clarendon Press, 1982.

Elizabeth I. *By the Queene. A proclamation against bringing in of wines or other merchandise from Bourdeaux, in respect of the plague being there*. 1585.

———. *By the Queen's Commandment. For as much as it is found by good proof that many persons which have served of late on the seas in the journey towards Spain and Portugal, in coming from Plymouth and other ports of the realm have fallen sick by the way and diverse died as infected with the plague*. 1589.

———. *Orders thought meete by her Maiestie, and her priuie Councell, to be executed throughout the Counties of this Realme, in such Townes, Uillages, and other places, as are, or may be hereafter infected with the plague, for the stay of further increase of the same. Also, an advise set downe upon her Majesties expresse commaundement, by the best learned in Physicke within this Realme, contayning sundry good rules and easie medicines, without charge to the meaner sort of people, as well for the preservation of her good Subjects from the plague before infection, as for the curing and ordring of them after they shalbe infected*. 1578.

———. *The Queenes most excellent Maiestie in her princely nature, considering how dangerous a matter it is by continuance of the faire called Bartholomew faire.* 1593.

Elyot, Sir Thomas. *The castel of helthe gathered, and made by Syr Thomas Elyot knight, out of the chief authors of phisyke; whereby euery man may knowe the state of his owne body, the preseruation of helthe, and how to instruct well his phisition in sicknes, that he be not deceyued.* 1539.

Erasmus. "Alchemy." In *Ten Colloquies,* edited by Craig R. Thompson, 47. New York: Liberal Arts Press, 1957.

———. *The Correspondence of Erasmus: Letters 142 to 297, 1501 to 1514.* Vol. 2. Translated by R. A. B. Mynors and D. F. S. Thomason. Toronto: University of Toronto Press, 1974.

———. *Oration in Praise of the Art of Medicine: Declamatio in laudem artis medicae.* In *Collected Works of Erasmus,* translated by Brian McGregor, 29:31–50. Toronto: University of Toronto Press, 1974.

Evelyn, John. *Fumifugium; or, The Inconveniencie of the Aer and Smoak of London Dissipated.* 1661.

Galen. *A Translation of Galen's Hygiene (De Sanitate Tuenda).* Translated by Robert Montraville Green. Springfield, Ill.: Charles C. Thomas, 1951.

Gasquet, Francie Aiden, and Edmund Bishop. *Edward VI and the Book of Common Prayer.* London: John Hodges, 1891.

Getz, Faye Marie. *Healing and Society in Medieval England: A Middle English Translation of the Pharmaceutical Writings of Gilbertus Anglicus.* Wisconsin Publications on the History of Science and Medicine 8. Madison: University of Wisconsin Press, 1991.

Greenblatt, Stephen. *Sir Walter Ralegh: The Man and His Roles.* New Haven, Conn.: Yale University Press, 1973.

Grigsby, Byron Lee. *Pestilence in Medieval and Early Modern English Literature.* New York: Routledge, 2004.

Grindal, Edmund. *The Remains of Edmund Grindal, Successively Bishop of London and Archbishop of York and Canterbury.* Edited by William Nicholson. Parker Society Publications 19. Cambridge: Cambridge University Press, 1968.

Healy, Margaret. *Fictions of Disease in Early Modern England: Bodies, Plagues, and Politics.* New York: Palgrave, 2001.

Helmstaedter, Gerhard. "Health Equilibrium of the Utopians on Well-Being and Hygiene." *Thomas Morus Jahrbuch, 1992*. Dusseldorf: Triltsh Verlag, 1993.

———. "Physicians in Thomas More's Circle: The Impact of the New Learning on Medicine." In *Thomas Morus Jahrbuch, 1989*, 158–64. Dusseldorf: Triltsch Verlag, 1989.

Henry VIII. "Limiting the Attendance at Baptism of Prince Edward." In *Tudor Royal Proclamations: Volume One, The Early Tudors (1485–1553)*, edited by Paul L. Hughes and James F. Larkin, Pages 259–60. New Haven, Conn.: Yale University Press, 1964.

Henshaw, Nathaniel. *Aero-chalinos; or, The Regifter for the Air; in Five Chapters*. Dublin: 1664.

Herford, C. H., Percy Simpson, and Evelyn Simpson, editors. *Ben Jonson*. 11 vols. Oxford, 1925–1952.

Herlihy, David. *Black Death and the Transformation of the West*. Cambridge: Harvard University Press, 1997.

Hexter, J. H. *More's Utopia: Biography of an Idea*. New York: Harper and Row, 1965.

Honan, Park. *Shakespeare: A Life*. Oxford: Oxford University Press, 1998.

Hooper, John. "Homily to be read in the time of Pestilence, 1563." In *Later Writings of Bishop Hooper*, edited by Charles Nevinson, 159–75. Parker Society Publications 52. Cambridge: Cambridge University Press, 1968.

Horrox, Rosemary, Editor and Translator. *Black Death*. Manchester Medieval Sources Series. Manchester: Manchester University Press, 1994.

Jacquart, Danielle. "Theory, Everyday Practice and Three Fifteenth-Century Physicians." In *Renaissance Medieval Learning: Evolution of a Tradition*, edited by Michael R. McVaugh and Nancy G. Siraisi, 140–60. Philadelphia: History of Science Society, 1991.

James I. *By the King Forasmuch as it hath pleased God of his exceeding goodnesse, to stay his heauy hand wherewith the last yeere hee punished our city of London by the infection of the plague*. 1604.

———. *Orders, thought meete by his Maiestie, and his Priuie Counsell, to be executed throughout the counties of this realme, in such townes, villages, and other places, as are, or may be hereafter infected with the plague, for the stay of further increase of the* same *by England and Wales.* 1603.

————. *Orders thought meet by His Maiestie, and his Priuy Councell, to bee executed throughout the counties of this realm, in such townes, uillages, and other places, as are, or may bee hereafter, infected with the plague, for the stay of further increase of the same also, An aduice set downe by the best learned physicke within this realme, containing sundry good rules and easie medicines, without charge to the meaner sort of people, as well for the preseruation of his good subjects from the plague before infection, as for the curing and ordering of them after they shall be infected.* 1625.

Janowitz, Henry D. "Helena's Medicine in All's Well That Ends Well: Is It Paracelsian or Hermetical in Origin?" *Cauda Pavonis: Studies in Hermeticism* 20:1 (2001): 20–22.

Jardine, Lisa. *Francis Bacon: Discovery and the Art of Discourse.* New York: Cambridge University Press, 1974.

Jonson, Benjamin. *The Alchemist.* Edited by Elizabeth Cook. The New Mermaids Series. London: A & C Black, 1991.

————. *The Complete Poetry of Ben Jonson.* Edited by William B. Hunter, Jr. Anchor Seventeenth-Century Series. Garden City, N.Y.: Doubleday, 1963.

————. *Volpone.* In *Elizabethan Plays,* edited by Hazelton Spencer, 299–352. Boston: Heath, 1933.

Jonson, Benjamin, George Chapman, and John Marston. *Eastward Ho,* edited by C. G. Petter. New Mermaids Series. London: Ernest Benn, 1973.

Jordan, Mark D. "The Construction of a Philosophical Medicine: Exegesis and Argument in Salernitian Teaching on the Soul." In *Renaissance Medieval Learning: Evolution of a Tradition,* edited by Michael R. McVaugh and Nancy G. Siraisi, 42–61. Philadelphia: History of Science Society, 1991.

Jordan, W. K. *Edward the Sixth: The Young King.* London: Allen and Unwin, 1968.

Kahn, Coppelia. "Magic of Bounty: *Timon of Athens,* Jacobean Patronage and Maternal Power." *Shakespeare Quarterly* 38:1 (1987): 34–57.

Karlen, Arlo. *Man and Microbes: Disease and Plagues in History and Modern Times.* New York: Putnam's, 1995.

Kay, W. David. *Ben Jonson: A Literary Life*. New York: St. Martin's, 1995.

Keller, Eve. "Producing Petty Gods: Margaret Cavendish's Critique of Experimental Science." *English Literary History* 64 (1997): 447–71.

Keller, James R. "Paracelsian Medicine in Donne's 'Hymn to God, My God, in My Sickness.'" *Seventeenth-Century News* 59:1–2 (2001): 154–58.

Kerrigan, William. *The Sacred Complex: On the Psychogenesis of Paradise Lost*. Cambridge, Mass.: Harvard University Press, 1983.

Kibre, Pearl. *Studies in Medieval Science: Alchemy, Astrology, Mathematics, and Medicine*. London: Hambledon Press, 1984.

Knight, G. Wilson. *The Wheel of Fire: Interpretations of Shakespearean Tragedy*. New York: Methuen, 1983.

Knoll, Robert E. *Ben Jonson's Plays: An Introduction*. Lincoln: University of Nebraska Press, 1964.

Knowles, Daniel, and R. Neville Hadcock. *Medieval and Religious Houses: England and Wales*. Great Britain: Longman, 1971.

Kreider, Alan. *English Chantries: The Road to Dissolution*. Cambridge, Mass.: Harvard University Press, 1979.

Leavy, Barbara Fass. *To Blight with Plague: Studies in a Literary Theme*. New York: New York University Press, 1992.

Le Guin, Ursula K. "The Ones Who Walk Away from Omelas." *Utopian Studies* 2:1–2 (1991): 1–5.

Lennard, John. *But I Digress: The Exploitation of Parentheses in English Printed Verse*. Oxford: Clarendon Press, 1991.

Leslie, Marina. *Renaissance Utopias and the Problem of History*. Ithaca, N.Y.: Cornell University Press, 1998.

Lev, Michael A. "Chinese Turn to Herbs to Root Out SARS." In *The Chicago Tribune*. http://www.apria.com/resources/1,2725,494-26998,00.html. Accessed April 11, 2003.

Lindberg, Carter. *European Reformations*. Cambridge, Mass.: Blackwell, 1996.

Lodge, Thomas. *A treatise of the plague containing the nature, signes, and accidents of the same, with the certaine and absolute cure of the feuers, botches and carbuncles that raigne in these times: and aboue all things most singular experiments and preseruatiues in the same, gathered by the obseruation of diuers worthy trauailers, and selected out of the writing of the best learned phisitians in this age. By Thomas Lodge, Doctor in Phisicke.* 1603

Londons Lamentation, or, A fit admonishment for City and Countrey, Wherein is described certaine causes of this affliction and visitation of the Plague, yeare 1641. 1641.

*Looking-glasse for city and countrey vvherein is to be seene many fearfull examples in the time of this grieuous visitation, with an admonition to our Londoners flying from the city, and a perswasion[to the?] country to be more pitifull to such as come for succor amongst them.*1630.

Lucian. *Timon; or, The Misanthrope.* In *Lucian of Samosata.* Vol. 2. Translated by A. M. Harmon. Loeb Classical Library. Cambridge, Mass.: Harvard University Press, 1913.

Lucretius. *De Rerum Natura.* 2 vols. Translated by W. H. D. Rouse. Loeb Classical Library. Cambridge, Mass.: Harvard University Press, 1996.

MacNalty, Arthur S. "Sir Thomas More as Public Health Reformer." In *Essential Articles for the Study of Thomas More,* edited by R. S. Sylvester and G. P. Marc'hadour, 119–36. The Essential Articles Series. Hamden, Conn.: Archon Books, 1977.

Mallin, Eric Scott. *Inscribing the Time: Shakespeare and the End of Elizabethan England.* Berkeley and Los Angeles: University of California Press, 1995.

Mandeville, John. *Mandeville's Travels.* Edited by M. C. Seymour. Oxford: Clarendon Press, 1967.

Marlowe, Christopher. *The Tragical History of Doctor Faustus.* In *Christopher Marlowe: Five Plays,* edited by Havelock Ellis, 41–63. New York: Hill and Wang, 1969.

Marshall, Louise. "Manipulating the Sacred: Image and Plague in Renaissance Italy." *Renaissance Quarterly* 47:3 (1994): 485–531.

Martin, A. Lynn. *Plague? Jesuit Accounts of Epidemic Disease in the Sixteenth Century.* Sixteenth Century Studies 28. Missouri: Sixteenth Century Journal, 1996.

Martin, Mathew. "Play and Plague in Ben Jonson's *The Alchemist.*" *English Studies in Canada* 26:4 (2000): 393–408.

May, Stephen. *Sir Walter Ralegh.* Twayne English Author Series. Boston: Twayne, 1989.

McCutcheon, Elizabeth. "William Bullein's Dialogue Against the Fever Pestilence: A Sixteenth-Century Anatomy." In *Miscellanea Moreana: Essays for Germain Marc'hadour*, edited by Clare M. Murphy, Henri Gibaud, and Mario A. Di Cesare, 341–59. Binghamton, N.Y.: Medieval and Renaissance Texts and Studies, 1989.

McVaugh, Michael R. *Medicine before the Plague: Practitioners and Their Patients in the Crown of Aragon, 1285–1345.* Cambridge: Cambridge University Press, 1993.

———. "The Nature and Limits of Medical Certitude at Early Fourteenth-Century Montpellier." In *Renaissance Medieval Learning: Evolution of a Tradition*, edited by Michael R. McVaugh and Nancy G. Siraisi, 62–85. Philadelphia: History of Science Society, 1991.

McVaugh, Michael R. and Nancy G. Siraisi, Editors. *Renaissance Medical Learning: Evolution of a Tradition.* Philadelphia: History of Science Society, 1991.

Miles, Rosalind. *Ben Jonson: His Life and Work.* New York: Routledge and Kegan Paul, 1986.

Milton, John. *Paradise Lost.* In *John Milton: Complete Poems and Major Prose*, edited by Merritt Y. Hughes. New York: Macmillan Publishing, 1957.

———. *The Reason of Church Government.* In *Complete Poems and Major Prose*, edited by Merritt Y. Hughes, 640–89. New York: Macmillan Publishing, 1957.

More, Thomas. *The Utopia.* In *The Complete Works of Thomas More*, vol. 4, edited by Edward Surtz and J. H. Hexter. New Haven, Conn.: Yale University Press, 1965.

———. *The Life of Pico.* In *The Complete Works of St. Thomas More*, vol. 1, edited by S. G. Anthony, Katherine Gardiner Rodgers, and Clarence H. Miller. New Haven, Conn.: Yale University Press, 1997.

Moylan, Tom. *Demand the Impossible: Science Fiction and the Utopian Imagination.* New York: Methuen, 1986.

———. *Scraps of the Untainted Sky: Science Fiction, Utopia, Dystopia.* Boulder, Colo.: Westview Press, 2000.

Mullett, Charles F. *The Bubonic Plague and England: An Essay in the History of Preventative Medicine.* Lexington: University of Kentucky Press, 1956.

Nashe, Thomas. *Christs teares ouer Ierusalem Wherunto is annexed, a comparatiue admonition to London.* 1593.

Neale, J. E. *Queen Elizabeth.* New York: Harcourt, Brace, 1934.

North, Sir Thomas, translator. "Life of Alcibiades." In *Plutarch's Lives of the Noble Grecians and Romans,* vol. 3. New York: AMS Press, 1967.

———. "Plutarch's Life of Marcus Antonius." In *Plutarch's Lives of the Noble Grecians and Romans,* vol. 6. New York: AMS Press, 1967.

Nugent, Elizabeth M., editor. *The Thought and Culture of the English Renaissance: An Anthology of Tudor Prose, 1481–1555.* Cambridge: Cambridge University Press, 1955.

Nutton, Vivian. "Humanist Surgery." In *The Medical Renaissance of the Sixteenth Century,* edited by A. Wear, R. K. French, and I. M. Lonie, 75–99. Cambridge: Cambridge University Press, 1985.

Oliver, Wade. *Stalkers of Pestilence: The Story of Man's Ideas of Infection.* Maryland: McGrath Publishing, 1970.

Olson, Glending. *Literature as Recreation in the Later Middle Ages.* Ithaca, N.Y.: Cornell University Press, 1982.

Orme, Nicholas and Margaret Webster. *The English Hospital 1070–1570.* New Haven, Conn.: Yale University Press, 1995.

Osler, William. *Thomas Linacre.* Cambridge: Cambridge University Press, 1908.

Pagel, Walter. *From Paracelsus to Van Helmont: Studies in Renaissance Medicine and Science,* edited by Marianne Winder. New York: Variorum Reprints, 1986.

———. *Paracelsus: An Introduction to Philosophical Medicine in the Era of the Renaissance.* Basel, Switzerland: S. Karger, 1958.

———. *The Religious and Philosophical Aspects of van Helmont's Science and Medicine.* Supplements to the Bulletin of the History of Medicine 2. Baltimore: The John Hopkins Press, 1944.

Palmer, R. "Pharmacy in the Republic of Venice in the Sixteenth Century." In *The Medical Renaissance of the Sixteenth Century,* edited by A. Wear, R. K. French, and I. M. Lonie, 100–117. Cambridge: Cambridge University Press, 1985.

Paré, Ambrose. *The workes of that famous chirurgion Ambrose Parey translated out of Latine and compared with the French. by Th. Johnson.* 1634.

Paris Medical Faculty. "The Report of the Paris Medical Faculty, October 1348." In *The Black Death,* translated and edited by Rosemary Horrox, 158–63. Manchester Medieval Sources Series. Manchester: Manchester University Press, 1994.

Peltonen, Markku, editor. *The Cambridge Companion to Bacon.* New York: Cambridge University Press, 1996.

Pollitzer, Robert. *Plague.* World Health Organization Monograph Series 22. Geneva: World Health Organization, 1954.

Ralegh, Sir Walter. *The Discovery of the Large, Rich, and Beautiful Empire of Guiana.* 1596. Edited by Robert Schomburgk. London: Printed for the Hakluyt Society, 1848.

Rawley, William. "To the Reader." In *The Works of Francis Bacon,* 14 vols., edited by James Spedding, Robert L. Ellis, and Douglas D. Heath, 2:335–37; 3:127. London: Longman, 1857–1874; rpt. New York: Garrett Press, 1968.

Reynolds, E. E. *The Field Is Won: The Life and Death of Saint Thomas More.* London: Burns and Oates, 1968.

Rogers, John. *The Matter of Revolution: Science, Poetry, and Politics in the Age of Milton.* Ithaca, N.Y.: Cornell University Press, 1996.

Ross, Cheryl. "The Plague of the Alchemist." *Renaissance Quarterly* 41:3 (1988): 439–57.

Rowse, A. L. *William Shakespeare: A Biography.* New York: Harper and Row, 1963.

———. *Shakespeare the Man.* Bristol: Western Printing Services, 1973.

Russel, Thomas. *Diacatholicon Aureum or A generall powder of Gold, purging all offensive humours in mans bodie.* 1602.

Sabine, Ernest L. "Butchering in Medieval London." *Speculum* 8:3 (1933): 335–53.

Samman, Neil. "The Progresses of Henry the Eighth: 1509–29." In *The Reign of Henry VIII: Politics, Policy and Piety,* edited by Diarmaid MacCulloch, 59–74. New York: St. Martin's, 1995.

Sargent, Lyman Tower. "The Three Faces of Utopianism Revisited." *Utopian Studies.* 5:1 (1994): 1–37.

———. "Utopian Traditions: Themes and Variations." In *Utopia: The Search for the Ideal Society,* edited by Rland Schaer, Gregory Claeys, and Lyman Tower Sargent, 8–15. New York: New York Public Library; Oxford: Oxford University Press, 2001.

Sargent, Rose-Mary. "Bacon as an Advocate for Cooperative Scientific Research." In *The Cambridge Companion to Bacon,* edited by Markku Peltonen, 146–71. Cambridge: Cambridge University Press, 1996.

Schaer, Roland, Gregory Claeys, and Lyman Tower Sargent, editors. *Utopia: The Search for the Ideal Society in the Western World.* New York: New York Public Library, 2001.

Schoenfeldt, Michael C. *Bodies and Selves in Early Modern England: Physiology and Inwardness in Spenser, Marlowe, Herbert, and Milton.* Cambridge: Cambridge University Press, 1999.

Schuler, Robert M. *Francis Bacon and Scientific Poetry.* Transactions of the American Philosophical Society 82.2. Philadelphia: American Philosophical Society, 1992.

———. "Jonson's Alchemists, Epicures, and Puritans." *Medieval & Renaissance Drama in England* 2 (1985): 171–208.

Seymour, M. C., editor. *Mandeville's Travels.* Oxford: Clarendon Press, 1967.

Shakespeare, William. *King Henry IV, Part 2.* Edited by A. R. Humphries. In *The Arden Shakespeare: The Complete Works,* 2nd ed., 393–428. London: Thomas Learning, 2001.

———. *Measure for Measure.* Edited by J. W. Lever. In *The Arden Shakespeare: The Complete Works,* 2nd ed., 801–30. London: Thomas Learning, 2001.

———. *Merry Wives of Windsor.* Edited by Giorgio Melchiori. In *The Arden Shakespeare: The Complete Works,* 2nd ed., 859–88. London: Thomas Learning, 2001.

———. *The Tempest.* Edited by Virginia Mason Vaughan and Alden T. Vaughan. In *The Arden Shakespeare: The Complete Works,* 2nd ed., 1071–96 London: Thomas Learning, 2001.

———. *Timon of Athens.* Edited by H. J. Oliver. In *The Arden Shakespeare: The Complete Works,* 2nd ed., 1097–1124. London: Thomas Learning, 2001.

Shrewsbury, J. F. D. *A History of Bubonic Plague in the British Isles.* Cambridge: Cambridge University Press, 1970.

Siraisi, Nancy. *Medieval and Early Renaissance Medicine: An Introduction to Knowledge and Practice.* Chicago: University of Chicago Press, 1990.

Slack, Paul. *The Impact of Plague in Tudor and Stuart England.* London: Clarendon Press, 1985.

———. Introduction to *Epidemics and Ideas: Essays on the Historical Perception of Pestilence*, edited by Terence Ranger and Paul Slack, 21–44. Past and Present Publications. Cambridge: Cambridge University Press, 1992.

Smith, Melissa. "The House, Sir, has been Visited: The Playhouse as Plaguehouse in Early Modern Revenge Tragedy." *The Journal of the Washington Academy of Science* 89: 1–2 (2003).

Soellner, Rolf. *Timon of Athens: The Pessimistic Tragedy*. Columbus: Ohio State University Press, 1979.

Steel, David. "Plague Writing from Boccaccio to Camus." *Journal of European Studies* 11:2 (1981): 88–110.

Stephens, James. *Francis Bacon and the Style of Science*. Chicago: University of Chicago Press, 1975.

Stow, John. *Survey of London*. 1603. 2 vols. Oxford: Clarendon Press, 1908.

Surtz, Edward and J. H. Hexter, editors. *The Utopia*. Vol. 4, *The Complete Works of Thomas More*. New Haven, Conn.: Yale University Press, 1965.

Summers, Claude J., and Ted-Larry Pebworth. *Ben Jonson*. Twayne English Author Series. New York: G. K. Hall, 1979.

Talbot, Charles. *Medicine in Medieval England*. London: Oldbourne, 1967.

Taylor, John. *The fearefull summer, or, Londons calamity, the countries courtesy, and both their Misery*. 1625.

Taylor, Steven M. "Portraits of Pestilence: The Plague in the Works of Machaunt and Boccaccio." *Allegorica* 5:1 (1980): 105–18.

Taylor, William F. *The Charterhouse of London: Monastery, Palace, and Thomas Sutton's Foundation*. London: J. M. Dent and Sons 1912.

Thomas, Keith. *Religion and the Decline of Magic*. New York: Scribner, 1971.

Totaro, Rebecca. "Plague and Promise: Golden Destinations and a 'Ship of Fools' during the English Renaissance." In *Reading the Sea: New Essays on Sea Literature*, edited by Kevin Alexander Boon, 175–84. New York: Fort Schuyler Press, 1999.

———. "Plague's Messengers: Communicating Hope and Despair in England, 1500–1700." *The Journal of the Washington Academy of Science* 89: 1–2 (2003).

United States Food and Drug Administration. "FTC and FDA Crackdown on Internet Marketers of Bogus SARS Prevention Products." In *FDA News.* http://www.fda.gov/bbs/topics/NEWS/2003/NEW00904.html. Available September 23, 2004.

Wager, William. *Enough Is as Good as a Feast: English Morality Plays and Moral Interludes,* edited by Edgar T. Schell and J. D. Shuchter, 367–418. New York: Holt, Rinehardt, and Winston, 1969.

Wear, A., R. K. French, and I. M. Lonie. Introduction to *The Medical Renaissance of the Sixteenth Century,* edited by A. Wear, R. K. French, and I. M. Lonie, ix–xvi. Cambridge: Cambridge University Press, 1985.

Webster, John. *The Duchess of Malfi.* Edited by Elizabeth M. Brennan. New Mermaids Series. New York: W. W. Norton, 1993.

Whitaker, Katie. *Mad Madge: The Extraordinary life of Margaret Cavendish, Duchess of Newcastle, the First Woman to Live by Her Pen.* New York: Basic Books, 2002.

Willard, Thomas. "Donne's Anatomy Lesson: Vesalian or Paracelsian?" *John Donne Journal: Studies in the Age of Donne* 3:1 (1984): 35–61.

Williams, Neville. *Henry the Eight and His Court.* London: Weidenfeld and Nicolson, 1971.

Wilson, F. P. *The Plague in Shakespeare's London.* 1927. Oxford: Oxford University Press, 1963.

World Health Organization. "Plague." http://www.who.int/health_topics/plague/en/. Avaliable September 22, 2004.

Wright, Louis B. *Gold, Glory and the Gospel: The Adventurous Lives and Times of Renaissance Explorers.* New York: Atheneum, 1970.

Zagorin, Peter. *Francis Bacon.* Princeton: Princeton University Press, 1998.

Index